I0085307

WHY WE DON'T ACHIEVE SH*T

Pasteur Tran

Copyright © 2020 by Pasteur Tran

mail@passytee.com
www.passytee.com

All rights reserved. No part of this publication may be reproduced, stored in retrieval system, copied in any form or by any means, electronic, mechanical, photocopying, recording or otherwise transmitted without written permission from the publisher. You must not circulate this book in any format.

The right of Pasteur Tran to be identified as author of this work has been asserted by him in accordance with sections 77 and 78 of the Copyright, Designs and Patents Act 1988.

Cover design by Adam Renvoize
Formatting by Polgarus Studio

Printed in the United States of America
First Edition

Contents

FRUSTRATED ACHIEVERS

I was sitting across from my friend at a café. He wasn't looking that great. He was well dressed, but he clearly was upset about something. After ordering a coffee, he looked at me and went straight into the reason he wanted to chat.

"I fucking hate my job, Pas. I want to quit."

This wasn't new. He has hated the *same* job every damn year. Every year, he would complain that he hated his job. Every year, he would go back to that job and work hard anyway.

It was an endless cycle.

Terry was one of those people who hated his job, wanted to quit, and was capable of so much more and he knew it. In fact, based on his CV alone, I'm sure he was more than qualified to run his own little business, which is what he wanted.

His work treated him like shit. Extended hours, with no extra pay.

He had a boss who demanded he do mundane tasks without letting him learn or grow in any sort of way. His friends told him to go out and do drugs.

Even having a coffee felt like a privilege because I never saw him unless he needed to vent.

"Well, Terry, you have always hated your job…" I stopped myself. To be honest, I was tired of him saying the same shit over and over again.

I decided to just tell him the truth.

"You won't quit your job, even though you hate the place. But let's be serious here, you keep saying you have no time to work on other projects. You sit and complain about shit, but never address them. You say you have toxic friends who consume the rest of your time. How do you plan to change your job, anyway?"

Once I stopped talking, he was shocked. I was shocked. All I was thinking was *"Fuck, was that too brutal?"*

The waiter served us our coffee and an eerie silence followed.

Terry stared at me. I could see he was tempted to fight back. He then stared at his coffee. Then, with a sudden jolt, looked up and said, "Fuck. You're right."

There are many people like Terry.

People capable of achieving amazing things—but they choose not to. From the guy who wants to start his own business but instead of starting he chooses to rework his plan over and over again, to the lady who can't write a book because she surrounds herself with toxic people. From the young man who just parties and doesn't care about tomorrow, to the lady who ignores opportunities because she recently broke up with her husband. The list is endless.

But who cares about them, right? What about *you*? Why don't you achieve what you want? Why are you choosing not to? What is holding you back?

I get frustrated with people who won't work to achieve their goals. If life has taught me anything, it's that you can achieve anything, *if* you put your mind to it.

Everyone is capable. Everyone has potential. You will hear excuses such as: *If only he tried a little harder. If only she would actually give it a sho*t. *Whether you realize your potential or not is completely up to you.*

In this book, I have distilled the reasons why people don't achieve the shit they want. In part, I wrote it out of frustration after seeing so many ridiculously skilled people wasting their time. They think they need motivation but can't see that there are different things that need to be addressed, such as fear, insecurity, or comparing themselves to the wrong people.

The main reason for writing this book, however, was to create a reference for people who need that extra push, because just saying "Go fucking achieve" doesn't always work. Yes, very selfish. But in reality, I want you to achieve what you want. It's satisfying knowing that reading this book might help you turn a corner in your life, that maybe this book is what makes you actually go achieve your goals. Upon reaching the end of it, I hope you believe that you *are* capable.

This book is organized in layers. The first layer is you.

You need to be in the right mental space or you aren't going to achieve shit. If you don't believe in yourself, you are screwed. If you are too scared to record your first video, because you want to be a YouTube star, then how the hell do you plan to achieve that? Just *hoping* it will come to you one day won't work. You must concentrate on you first.

The second layer is about your goal.

We are in a society where people seem to judge and pull you down. They tell you your goal is shit, or not worthwhile. How you plan to achieve your goal is discussed here.

Do you refuse to set a deadline? Or do you hope that your goal will just happen by pure luck? Or perhaps you're working with goals that aren't even yours.

If you answered yes, then you aren't motivated; you really don't even fucking care. This layer addresses why people don't achieve their goals.

The final layer is the people around you. The people who will support you in obtaining your dreams.

Are the people around you toxic? Or are they cheerleaders hoping to see you succeed? Some people will stab you in the back. Others will, out of charity, help you and push you in the right direction. Who you surround yourself with is important. This layer is about the factors that influence you externally.

By the end of this book, I want you to be able to realize you are capable of achieving goals by seeing the reasons people fail to get the shit they want.

You deserve to live your dreams. You can do it. Some people are born lucky, others just have it better than you, but no one has the same path for the same goal.

Goals are unique. If you want to be a writer, an actor, a dentist, a vlogger—it doesn't matter—you *can* achieve what you want.

I see so many amazing people failing to get what they want; I hope you can learn from their mistakes and pursue your dreams.

Everyone in this book is real, but I have changed their names and professions to keep things private. I am thankful for everyone who has influenced me and helped me create this book.

Now, let's get to it, achiever…

PART I

YOU

You are the single constant in your life.
So, it is on *you* to achieve.

1. YOU DON'T TAKE SHOTS

There's a cliché that has always bugged me: "You can't win the lottery unless you buy a ticket." I thought it was a way for a gambler to justify his gambling addiction. I don't have a chance to win money so I *must* buy a ticket.

But life is just like that. You don't get a chance for success unless you play.
You can't achieve shit unless you buy a ticket.

I remember walking into my friend's five-bedroom, five-bath mansion on the 54th floor. It was certainly an amazing sight. But a question gnawed at me, so I asked.

"Kenny, how much does this place cost? Only if you're comfortable telling me, of course, because this is fucking huge."

He didn't flinch. "$12.5 million USD."

My gut reaction was simply awe. But then, something really started to eat at me. *How do I afford a place like this?* Doing quick math in my head, I would need a smooth $2 million alone, just to have a deposit on the mortgage. I didn't need to calculate how much I would owe the bank on a monthly basis; the first barrier was the damn $2 million cash.

Who just has that in the bank?

Kenny was a risk taker. His parents didn't make a lot, and he grew up thinking money was everything. He worked odd jobs when I was probably playing Mario Kart on my Super Nintendo.

Kenny was always taking shots.

When he had an idea, he would do it. The idea didn't have to be great, it just simply had to exist. When we were young and playing Pokémon cards, we thought of making our own collectable card game. We brought a printer and started designing cards. Realistically, we just copied the entire concept of Pokémon cards and changed the pictures and themes. We printed our cards out and started selling them to other students. It's amazing what you can do when you are young. We didn't care if you didn't buy them because we felt other kids would. We made some nice cash. We had no idea about cash flow and accounting. The idea gave us money and we loved it. But then Pokémon and any other form of trading cards were banned from school because kids were caught stealing from each other.

Business closed.

But Kenny's natural entrepreneurial spirit didn't stop. He would run with ideas whenever he could. Once, he had a string of bad ideas: custom-made shirts, followed by a board game, and then topped off with a magnetic calendar for the fridge. Each one failed. Each idea was executed and thrown into a pile of bad ideas.

Life eventually starts to catch up and you can't afford to keep taking shots.

Kenny fell in love and got married. He had to find a stable job, and that's exactly what he did.

I thought that was the end of the story. It wasn't.

After all, as I stood there in his mansion it was obvious that Kenny couldn't afford his ridiculous mansion if he all he took was a stable job. As it happens, he kept taking little shots every year. Perhaps not large gambles but he still tried out different ideas.

Kenny had invested in a little mobile application company. The iPhone was announced and a surge in demand for mobile apps grew. When the iPhone first came out, almost any decent application would be a hit. Running through a string of successful hits, Kenny made it big.

He sold his shares and he made money. A lot of it. Enough to buy the mansion outright. But when I talked to him about how he knew what to invest in, he had no clue. He had a sense that apps might be the future, but with no certainty was he right. He achieved his goal—to make a fuck-load of money—by taking a shot.

I've always wondered what would happen if I told you that Kenny just invested in a business and got lucky. He *did* get lucky. But luck only comes to those who actually choose to play. The more shots you take, the more chance one will work. But there's also a chance that none of them will work.

On the other hand, there are people who are lucky first thing—and that's just how the game goes. It is *possible* that someone buys a lottery ticket for the first time and wins.

Possible, but unlikely.

A colleague of mine, Sam, was also a person who took shots.

He was very inspirational, and certainly made me believe in always going with any opportunity that is given to you. Sam had started a successful beauty clinic and skincare company. Before that, he had tried drop-shipping skincare and investing in natural skincare boutiques in Australia.

These first ideas failed, but he picked himself up and finally took over a small store in Melbourne. He put in natural cosmetic products and started growing a little boutique.

But like Kenny, life comes up with crazy surprises. For Sam, he unfortunately was diagnosed with cancer. Sam decided to sell his business in bits and pieces to the highest bidder. He now enjoys a simple life in a country town of Australia.

He never got to cash in his lottery ticket. You can take shots and one finally hits. You can take shots and they may never hit. If you want to achieve something in your life, you have to take risks.

Life is ultimately about deciding whether you want to play.

If you want a "normal" life, it makes sense to take fewer shots. You should follow a safe path. There is nothing wrong with that. Shots are costly. You either spend time, or money—and probably both. You could drain your resources into one shot and it fails.

Tread the steady life or choose to play.

The most important thing is knowing that you may lose. Others, who may seem undeserving, may still win. But that is what a game is.

Lucky breaks come to those who play. If you sit on the sideline, you can't get lucky, because you aren't in the game. So, to achieve what you want, play—and play hard.

2. YOU COMPLAIN WITH NO ACTION

Don't you love complaining?

"I hate my job. I want to quit." "I hate my house.... it's so small."

So, why don't you change things?

You complain because, inside, you know that something is better. You know something better *does* exist. And somewhere inside, you must know that you are capable of achieving it. You know it's possible.

You complain about what you can get, not what you can't.

When you fall over, why don't you complain about gravity? It's gravity's fault that you fell over and hurt your leg. Why aren't you cursing to the world that gravity is the most stupidest thing ever?

When have you heard someone complain that water sucks? Or leaves are too green? Or what about the fact that milk is white. Damn that milk!

It's not possible to complain about these things because they're not changeable. They are facts. You can't do anything about it, so you *can't* complain.

For things that you can change, if you complain and don't do anything about it, you're only hurting yourself. You're reminding yourself you *can* do something about your situation—a better job or perhaps a better car—but are *choosing* not to do anything.

By the time you decide to start, it's going to be too late. Stop complaining and actually do something about it.

Get on with your goals in your life as soon as you can.
The complaining is getting you nowhere.

I remember a guy who told me he hated his job. He didn't do a single thing about it, much like Terry at the beginning of this book. A few years later, he would still say he hated his job. No one wanted to be around him.

It's fine to initially complain because your complaint is a clear signal to what your goal should be. Imagine if your friend kept telling you that he hated his job every time you caught up. Soon, you wouldn't want to hear about it ever again. It would probably be far more interesting if he actually *did* complain about gravity. That way you would get a good laugh at the same time.

Now, think of the person who's working on a solution and wants to take action on what they dislike. She complains about her job, but she's actively seeking a new one. She starts to shape the future that she wants and, instead of complaining, she works on a path to address her own complaints. It is respectable and admirable, and she is someone we can look up to.

Years later, you might catch up for a drink and she might tell you, "I ended up quitting that job and started a business." That is amazing. That is something to be proud of. That is what you should be doing when you have a complaint: addressing the complaint head on.

It was 2017 when I did meet someone who told me he had quit his job. He had studied medicine and was five years post-graduation. He hated it. His parents made him pursue medicine and he was completely over it. It was not easy for him to quit, but he did. He moved into corporate finance and he's never been happier. It took him four years to plan it out and make the transition, but he fucking did it.

I had many questions for him. *How the fuck did you pivot from medicine to finance? Why on earth would you do that? What about all those wasted years studying?*

But all I ended up asking was, "Are you enjoying it?"

His answer was a resounding *yes*.

He told me how much he had always wanted it. He didn't want to just sit around and complain, so he set his mind on doing finance and went with it. Seeing that you're probably curious, he acquired an MBA while working as a doctor to make a living. *To stop the complaining, he addressed what he was complaining about.*

Every time you have a complaint, think about how you can solve it. What's the core problem? If you're complaining about your job, work on getting a new job. If you're complaining that a subject is too damn hard, find a way to make it easier. If you complain about how someone is making so much money, find another job to make more money.

Complaints are the perfect indicator of what you should be working on.

I get it. Complaining is addictive. It feels so damn good to release that pent-up stress and aggravation. People will listen to you complain and they will also feel like they helped you by lending an ear.

But you don't *achieve* shit if all you do is complain. It's opportunity wasted. The time you spend complaining is time lost for working on your goals. Imagine if everyone just stood around and complained. We wouldn't have cars. We wouldn't have social media. We wouldn't have shit.

Let the rest of the world complain. You got shit to do.

But what if you're too scared to address the problem?

Maybe it's an internal complaint running around your mind. The problem is you will hear that complaint every day. And every day that shit will eat at you till you feel helpless.

I've been there.

I was too scared to tell my boss he should stop treating me like a doormat. Eventually, the complaint in my mind went away, but in the end that only happened because I started to accept his rudeness and his propensity to use me like a metaphorical doormat.

The option is simple: Address your complaint or don't complain.

Addressing your complaints can take courage. Doing so might risk losing your job or something else (spouse, friend, family member). But if you don't take the risk, you will simply continue complaining and stay miserable. Be brave. You might get a result that's better off for you.

Don't be the person who gets nothing done but seems to find the energy to complain. That's not to say you can't complain. Just write your complaint down, identify the goal within it, and figure out how you can go after it. Force it into simply being a problem that requires a solution. You know a solution exists; otherwise, the complaint would have never crossed your mind.

To achieve what you want you must address your complaints because they are the flashing signs around your true goals.

3. YOU PROCRASTINATE

What if I told you that if you don't clean your room you will die?

I was tired of the years you left it so dirty, so I decided to put a gun to your head. Going to clean the room now? You sure will. You had no reason to clean it before but, when your life is at stake, you will clean it as fast as humanly possible.

And why didn't you clean it before?

The answer is: tomorrow.

Tomorrow is so certain. We are living longer and longer. It's true; tomorrow *will* come for most of us.

But that's the problem. How can you be so sure? One day a plane may crash. When I wrote this chapter, Boeing had recently grounded its new planes due to two crashes.

Another day, a car accident may happen. You might get hit by some idiot *texting*! We are so sure about tomorrow coming that we become lazy. It's that very certainty that gives us a reason to procrastinate. The fact that you *know* you can do something later helps you convince yourself that it's okay you didn't get anything done today.

It's fine, I can do it tomorrow. I can do it next week. I can do it next year. Bam. You're dead. I know, it sounds very dark.

But we haven't found the elixir of life yet, have we?

So, what the hell does this have to do with achievement?

Well, it should make you realize that time can be cut short without your consent. You have no idea when it may happen and all you will remember is that you sat there procrastinating. You have a set time to do what you want in your life. The older you get, the harder it gets.

That's not to say you can't do things when you're older, it's just logistically harder. True, KFC was started when Colonel Sanders was in his 50s. Yes, Ray Kroc was also in his 50s when he decided to start McDonalds. But they are outliers. The older you get, the more risk adverse you become. You have got to work on what you want *now*.

This, however, is not a Y.O.L.O. (you only live once) Moment. People have taken this the wrong way. No, don't go spending your life savings without a plan. Don't go out drinking like crazy because you might die tomorrow.

This is to emphasize that if you want to achieve something amazing you won't have forever. The younger you are, the higher your chance of actually achieving what you set for yourself. So, why aren't you on the path to achieve the things you've always wanted? Why are you sitting at home doing absolutely nothing? What happened to those life goals that you wanted to pursue?

When I started to write this book, there was an article about a man who was stuck in a traffic jam and missed his flight. He was angry. He was upset. Damn, now he has to pay more money because he missed a flight. Guess what? His flight ended up crashing and there were no survivors. Lucky guy, huh?

When I hear these stories, I think about the times I have sat there doing absolutely nothing. I hear of people going out to achieve amazing things like climbing a ridiculously high mountain, jumping from space, or finishing a marathon in spectacular time.

"What have I been doing with my life?" is what I ask myself.

A meteor could hit the world. Lightning can strike at any moment. Windows have fallen from hotel rooms and claimed lives. You never know.

So, get on that path now. I'd rather die knowing I achieved the goals on my list, or at least started ticking them off, than to sit on a toilet bowl reading social media.

Perhaps you want to leave a legacy? By definition, no one gets to enjoy their legacy. If you want to achieve something after death, then you do you. There's a famous painter who was considered a madman in his lifetime and labeled a failure. He was also very poor. His paintings are now worth millions. His name? Vincent Van Gogh.

Did he get to enjoy that in his life? No.

In your life, you need to achieve your goals and enjoy them. Legacy will come by default from your achievements, but that can only be left if you achieve.

So, even if your goal is to leave a legacy, how do you plan to do that by procrastinating? Be remembered as the person who didn't even try? Better to be remembered as the person who did their best to get what they want.

You decide…

So, you really want to make that computer game? Go learn to code, *now.* Want to learn that language? Download the textbook, *now.* Maybe you want to study for that MBA? Maybe you want to change careers? The whole damn point is you start *now.*

Get on that road and go. No more idling. You need to start as soon as you can before it's too late.

> *Death is inevitable. Achieving what you want is questionable. The difference is you can control the latter. Time is limited. Don't waste it.*

4. YOU LACK AMBITION
AND GET SHOT DOWN

I'm surprised by how many people lack ambition. The most capable people can tell you about some vision they have or some idea they want to pursue—but do nothing about it. The moment you encourage them to pursue it, they lock up. They freeze. They seem to think they can't do it or convince themselves it's not worth it.

The dream ends.

When my friend said she wanted to study nursing and open a beauty clinic, I was pumped. I *knew* she would succeed. She had the right personality and flare to pull it off. She told me the fine details: how the spa would look, the style she would serve customers, and what would differentiate her business from other regular spas. She was going to make it. We talked about great locations and we looked at the fastest way to obtain her nursing degree. I couldn't wait to see her make it happen.

Five months later, I decided to message her and ask how the nursing degree was going. "I'm not doing it anymore," was her response. I was shocked.

I met up with her later in the week and it dawned on me that she convinced herself it was too hard. *I don't think I can do it. It's too much.* She shot herself down before she even started.

No matter how much I tried to convince her that it would work, she wouldn't budge. I was confident in her and was willing to invest my own money into her project.

But she was able to rationalize why she shouldn't and couldn't do it. It is very easy to throw ambition out the window. What she wanted to achieve was so easily discarded.

When I thought of her for this chapter, I messaged her to meet for a coffee. It had been a few years after our first meeting. She is still a receptionist. Her life hasn't changed at all.

"I wish I studied nursing," she would tell me.

I was crushed but told her she made the right choice.

I lied.

I do hope she reads this chapter and realizes that she still can obtain what she wants. Doing anything worthwhile is scary. We suppress our ambitions because we're worried about situations that haven't even happened.

You can't become successful if you don't light that
small bit of fiery ambition inside of you.

Why bother dreaming at all? Why bother creating a fantasy world for yourself if you aren't willing to take the shot? You only hurt yourself. You build a beautiful house inside your mind only to crush it.

People all have visions but, with time, they continually beat them down or let others smash away at them. Then they regret what they didn't do.

You should only pursue ambition if it's in you. And because you picked up this book, I know that it's in you.

Some people are unlucky. They never had anyone or anything supporting them to help them believe they can achieve more. I have more than a handful of friends who are happy to live a simple life and complain about dreams that *feel* unattainable. That's not you, that's them—and this book is about *you*.

I have pushed friends to pursue their dreams and goals. Oddly enough, I have lost friends because I did so. They felt like I was too much. I was pushing my own agenda onto them.

You don't need to push your ambitions and goals onto other people. You don't even need to be upset about it either. I know I have in the past. I say this because much like my friend and her nursing goals, I had pushed her too hard and got caught up in the moment. I knew she was capable, but she chose not to pursue it. That's her loss, not mine.

Instead of helping other people, concentrate on finding things to support your dreams.

Are you actually being a good friend if you don't push your friends to do what they are capable of? Not really. It's simply not worth it.

When I pushed a friend to start his own photography company, he gave up. When I pushed a friend to purse an online personal training platform, he kept going. What was the difference? One was already on the path; the other hadn't even started.

If you want to support people, look for ambitious people who have *already* started on their goals. For the rest, just let them be and let them work out what they want.

I realized that the reason I pushed people was because I wanted the support of other ambitious people. If I couldn't find them I would instill it upon others.

But that's not how it works. People need to find their own ambition first.

You must work on you first. Truly ask what you want to achieve and create a map toward it. Don't let anyone affect your initial decisions. If you believe you deserve and can obtain your goal, create a loose idea on how you plan to get there. Maybe you want to get those big biceps. So, plan what exercises you need to do and what you need to eat to build muscle.

Ambition is simply the pursuit of something greater. It doesn't have to be money or a fancy house. Heck, I think creating an orphanage in Cambodia is an extremely ambitious goal. If you told me you planned to build a 3,000-piece Lego set without instructions, I would think that's an ambitious goal—and good luck with that. If you have dreams or a visualization on who you want to be, that is ambition. That is what you should tap into as much as you can. *That* is part of how you achieve your goals.

Jasmine was a friend of mine who never tapped into her ambition. She is a physiotherapist specializing in women's health. She was brought up by parents who told her that she was "fine" and shouldn't do anything else and to just stay the course.

Although she had ambitions to open her own clinic, her parents thought otherwise. Every time her idea came to mind, her parents shut it down. *You are doing well. Look at everyone else your age! The economy is bad! It's a bad sign!* There was always a reason for her not to do it.

Her friend soon opened a clinic and asked her to join. She joined and helped grow the clinic. When the owner wanted to step away, Jasmine was offered to buy the clinic and own it completely.

But she said no. She would say that she was getting old. It wasn't the right time. It was as if ambition felt wrong to her. She stayed in the company and it expanded. She kept missing out and she soon became bitter. I have no doubt Jasmine is content at what she is doing. But on the other hand, I'm sure it's eating at her day in and day out knowing the company could have been hers.

You are capable of achieving and pursuing what you want. But, and this is a big but, you are far more capable of suppressing your ambition.

You have ambition. You have goals. You have dreams. Pursue them. There is no other option. We can't weigh the cost of regret till it's far too late.

You can't achieve shit if you shoot it down before it's even started.

5. YOU ARE SCARED OF FAILURE

No one can tell you that failure or rejection feels good, because it doesn't. It feels like shit. Failure can be as small as attempting to bake a red velvet cake and it ends up looking like Spam (and tastes like it, too). It could be asking someone out for a date and getting rejected. It could be pitching your idea to a bunch of venture capitalists and being told you should just quit.

Who the fuck would want that feeling?

To actually achieve shit, you *need* to fail.

When you get rejected for the first time, what happens? You are unsure what to do. You might even shed a tear or complain to your friends. You feel like crap. But, the next day, you wake up and you realize something. You are fucking alive! You have survived what felt like the end of the world. You are able to look back and see how you can improve.

What will stop you being rejected next time? Did you say something wrong? Maybe it was the spinach in your teeth. You learn. You may get rejected a hundred times after, but each time is a lesson that leads you toward achieving your goal.

Perhaps you want to pitch your idea to a few investors. Maybe your book is going to be the next best seller. Maybe you want to become a Twitch streamer and make fuck-loads of money. Whatever it may be, each goal requires you to fail. Nothing will go perfectly, and if it does, you just got damn lucky.

Look at comedians who go out and perform in front of an audience that boos them off stage. Even if the night before was shit, they *still* go out the next day and perform. Even if oranges get thrown at them or the night is quiet without a single laugh, they keep going.

That is what sets achievers apart. They wake up the day after a failure knowing they are still alive. They keep trying. It may feel horrible, but they go on.

But some people hold onto these bad feelings. Even though it's passed, they keep remembering their failures. All you should do is learn from them. Otherwise, you're digging into past failures that will only pull your down, convincing yourself that you will fail again. You don't want that feeling again. No one does.

If reliving your failures is what's stopping you, do you really think you will obtain your goals and dreams? Do you deserve to achieve shit if you aren't willing to fail? Have you convinced yourself that you should just stop so you will never feel failure again?

Just consider this: Realistically, you are failing yourself if you allow regret and a "what if" to gnaw away at you. *That* failure will last forever.

There are many people who won't move on from their failures. They will be haunted by some monumental failure and it will prevent them from achieving and reaching their potential.

A colleague of mine, David, was scarred from his first piano performance in front of an audience. That event was plagued with unlucky circumstances. A little boy in the audience was crying and his mother was desperately trying to put him to sleep. To make matters worse, it was customary to be suited and well dressed, but because the air conditioning was not working well, it made all the performers sweat bullets profusely.

When it was David's turn, he was not in a good state. Even when he went up to bow to the crowd, sweat was dripping off his forehead. He slipped on the keys and made horrible mistakes; it was almost a relief for him to finish the piece. He bowed once more and ran behind the curtains.

And that was it.

David would never touch a piano again. In fact, he would never want to perform for an audience in general. He had a natural talent. In classes, he was unparalleled and he always wanted to be a famous pianist. But from one small failure, he couldn't move on. He could no longer achieve what he wanted.

That isn't to say you can't be upset about failure. As I said before, it feels like shit. I hate the feeling, even though I've been rejected by countless numbers of people in relationships and in business.

There are high achievers who still feel horrible after failing: Steve Jobs, Marc Cuban, Kevin Hart, and Sam Walton to name a few. But they minimize the time they are upset. They don't let it scar them. Instead, they use that failure as a lesson.

That is how they achieved their goals. They saw failures for what they really are: lessons. Failures are for you to figure out how to succeed. They are hints for you to figure out what to do next. If you are feeling like crap about failure, think of it as a lesson and a step closer toward your goal.

Failure is never-ending. You can't avoid it if you plan to achieve. So … don't. If you plan to be successful, you must plan to fail. It will feel like the world is ending at first, but you will brush yourself off and get back up. And each time you do, you make failure easier.

Don't let failure have its way with you.

6. YOU BELIEVE IN WORK-LIFE BALANCE

"You just have to work harder. Fewer breaks and more work," I told my friend. He was offended. He had recently started a second-hand bookstore and his sales were flatlining.

"What do you mean I have to work harder? I'm doing the best I can!" he yelled at me. I was glad we were in an empty bar because anyone could have heard his booming voice.

"You aren't doing your best," I responded.

He was getting visibly angry. And rightly so. If someone came in and told you that you weren't doing your best when you *believed* you were, you would get very defensive.

"Look at it this way, how many hours do you play games, sleep, go out to eat, etcetera?" I asked.

He looked at me in disgust. "Those are times I need to relax and chill, man. Sometimes you need a balance in life."

That word—balance—is bullshit.

Do you think high achievers have long tea breaks? McDonald's, Apple, Microsoft, Virgin: Do you think the founders had a work-life balance? Absolutely not. They worked their asses off. They didn't have large breaks. Most of their hours were spent concentrating on building their business.

In order to achieve something, you must take your efforts to the extreme ends. Not to the middle because *nothing* happens in the middle. That is akin to putting in 50% effort and complaining you couldn't obtain your goals.

We would have a fuck load of achievers if people could afford time to relax while building their company, writing their book, or filming a successful movie.

You must put in excessive hours. You have to put in ridiculous dedication. Doesn't sound good, does it? But that is how you achieve shit. Not this bullshit work-life balance.

Work on your dreams as much as possible. Tilt the balance toward your actual goal as far as you can handle. To do that, you must sacrifice some of the luxuries you have.

We invented weekends. We invented breaks. We invented social media and video games. Heck, does anyone know where the whole eight hours of sleep was invented?

A lot of people will get angry hearing this. They fight back by saying they need their breaks.

I remember a teacher arguing with me that she needed to relax after a long day of work. Look, I get it. People have tough days. But this is about achieving shit, and if the only time you have to work on your other goals is in your breaks, well, *that's* where you are going to find the time.

Other people will point to science and say that you need to have rest! Somewhere on the Internet an article will tell you what you need to hear. After spending one minute on Google, I was able to find an article that said by spending *less* time doing shit I could achieve amazing things. What the fuck?

I once worked with a developer who was extremely talented. Once the clock hit 5 P.M., it was break time: a long session of gaming. Four to five hours of gaming, to be exact. He told us he needed it to de-stress.

Nothing wrong with that, it was his balance.

But one day over drinks he told all of us that he was annoyed he couldn't make his own game, that the company was taking all his time.

This sent one of the other developers off the rails. "You fucking play games every other hour, how can you say you don't have time?"

He argued that he needed to play games to give himself time to "re-calibrate."

You don't have the right to complain that you have no time when you sit around consuming entertainment instead of producing the stuff you want.

The reality is that some projects need more time than others. Some people don't need the same amount of time as you do. The larger your goal, the harder you must push yourself.

Work-life balance was an excuse made for people who wanted more time to rest. If you can afford to do so, why wouldn't you? If you can afford to have a lot of breaks and still achieve what you want, then go for it. That's an amazing luxury to have.

But most of us can't afford do to that. It is not a great feeling to admit you have to work hard to get what you want. No one wants to cut into the luxuries they have earned. You may have worked your ass off to get an expensive car, only to be told to sell it so you can fund your next venture. You could be told the next day you won't have any more free time to spend with your family, even though for years you worked hard to get that free time.

But achievement does come at a cost. So, are you willing to pay the price?

"How much do you want it?" I have asked some people. Most of the time, the answer is somewhere along the lines of "more than anything in this world." Yet, when you tell them to make the time, they lock up and get defensive. They don't want to give up the things they enjoy.

When my game company was nearing bankruptcy, I realized I still had time to go out and party. I was hanging out with friends and drinking. How was I going to achieve anything? You come to a realization that you aren't doing everything you can; you are the reason things are failing. I had to go into hermit mode. I started to spend more time with my developers and we were able to ship our first successful game.

Work-life balance is an excuse.

To achieve whatever it is that you want, you must find a balance that is suited to your specific goal. If you require a lot of time, then you will have to give up a lot of your luxury and free time. The bigger and more ambitious the goal, the less time you get for yourself. The further you are behind, the more you have to give up.

Suck it up. The only way for you to achieve the shit you want is to put absolutely everything you can into it.

There is no universal balance—only the one that works for you.

7. YOU LACK DISCIPLINE

Discipline is the one skill everyone can learn. If you are disciplined, you can achieve whatever goal you set yourself. Want to save money? You need to be disciplined. Want to be fit and healthy? Well, you're going to need that willpower to stop you from eating those snacks, and that involves discipline.

To be disciplined means to be in control.

I remember years of trying to lose weight. I failed every time. I could never lose the weight. I started really strong and was filled with energy, but after a while, I fizzled. That's how unforgiving discipline is as a muscle. If you don't use it, it's going to shrink faster than it takes for you to grow it. It is a habit you must work on forever.

Maintenance of your discipline is an ongoing struggle; you must maintain it until you die. Without discipline you cannot achieve your goals.

The beautiful part about discipline is that it's universal.

When you succeed in one goal—because you were dedicated and put in hard work toward getting a result—it seeps through to other facets in your life.

Athletes, content creators, authors, and pro gamers all need a form of discipline. If you put time into training for a marathon and you complete that marathon, you reinforce the fact that dedication pays off. So, if you put in time to learn chess, you could master it with enough time.

You build that muscle to work for other parts of your life.

If you can sit and program for hours to produce something to show your friends, you start to see that *doing* actual shit produces something tangible.

This was what my friend Steven did. He made a small multi-player game in his free time and hosted a small get-together. It was a simple concept: a bunch of mini-games. It was all the games we particularly loved to play when we were younger (like a fast-paced Mario Party for those gamers out there). It was fun and a great night. He then went on to improve the game and, a few months later, he added more games and improved the graphics.

He remained disciplined. Even during those boring nights tweaking the game, typing tedious code or fixing bugs, he made something we could all play and enjoy.

Steven quickly moved on and started working on an app he had always wanted to make. The thing is, he was always able to do it. What he lacked was discipline. Now, however, he had gained confidence and realized that his goal of making his own app was possible. Although I can't go into much detail, his app used images to recognize fashion items you might want to buy; finding clothing you are interested in online.

Discipline shows you that any goal is possible.

That is the magic of discipline. By seeing the results that Steven could obtain by dedicating himself to making a game for friends, he built the discipline to work on developing an app of his own.

Discipline is an amazing universal trait.

Every time you successfully gain results through hard work and discipline, a simple but effective feedback loop is created. Discipline gives you results. More results build more discipline. When you prove to yourself that discipline results in something good, that feedback is priceless.

My first discipline "result" was a small app I created for the iPhone. When I planned the app, it was simple map program. Once I finally built the app, I *felt* I could do more. I saw the *results* of sitting down without distractions, working on a project till I got it to do what I wanted, and persevering through the hard and boring times. I was building my muscle. This helped me build more apps, and although some weren't successful, I was able to build my own portfolio of self-made programs.

Something should be said about breaks and discipline.

I have heard countless times that you need breaks. Yes, taking breaks can allow your discipline to grow. Any training couch will tell you it's bad for you if you go to the gym every day. But as mentioned in the previous chapter, you need to find the balance that works for you.

It's an odd thing, but you can build discipline by controlling your breaks. I find it hard to just stick to exactly "fifteen minutes" or not binging on another episode of my favorite show while I'm relaxing.

So, discipline your breaks. If you can control your breaks, then your discipline grows. But if you prolong those breaks, which I have done, you ruin everything you worked on. I am guilty of watching that extra TV show, partying for far longer than I should have, or playing "one more" video game. Don't do this because if you do, regret will be waiting for you.

To achieve shit, you must grow that discipline. Set clear incremental goals and achieve them. Create that positive feedback loop. Perhaps you want to learn a language. Set a goal to learn one new phrase by the end of the week. Then break down the steps to achieving that phrase, what words will you need to learn and how much time you will dedicate to it.

Every goal requires discipline. It doesn't matter if you plan to become the best break-dancer or a cabinetmaker. You have to have discipline. It's a muscle that you *always* build. The more you relax and stop working on your projects or on yourself, the harder it will be to get back into it. It is far easier to relax than to actually achieve the shit you've wanted.

When things get hard, you have to remember that discipline muscle. You don't want it to get saggy and become nothing. Stick to the damn goal and get it done. Build that muscle till it's huge. Let your self-discipline pour into other facets of your life.

8. YOU WASTE FLASHES OF INSPIRATION

Have you ever had a flash of inspiration? A great idea, a sudden surge of energy that says, *I should really do this.* The best inspirations seem to happen at the most inconvenient times. I've woken up in the middle of the night in a cold sweat with a great idea (well, at least what I think is a great idea). I tell myself I'm going to start working on the idea when I wake up. I go back to sleep, and when I wake up, it's gone.

Good ideas come and go. You might be sitting on the toilet or in the shower. Heck, my friend told me her idea to open a cupcake store in Australia happened when she was scrolling through Pinterest in the bathroom.

Those are flashes of inspiration, and you need to capitalize on them when they happen.

Let's be honest though, if you were in the shower, you won't be making calls to set up a business. I would certainly not encourage you to leave your child's dance recital and start writing a book.

But inspiration can and does occur at random and inconvenient times. What's worse, we sabotage ourselves by doing something else, thinking we can act on our inspiration later. We play with our mobile phone. We spend time on the computer. We chat on Facebook. You *might* not forget the idea, but what about that extra energy? What about that immediate sudden surge of urgency? It's gone. *That* is what you need to use.

The best action is to force yourself onto the next step.

If all of a sudden you feel an urge to study Japanese, either buy a textbook online or enroll into an online course *right now*. There is a vast amount of material that is free, so you can start straight away.

Maybe you have a great business idea? Fuck yeah! What's the next step you can do? *It doesn't have to be huge, but it has to commit you to the idea.* Perhaps you want to make cakes. Buy the recipe book or the utensils to cook *now*. Invite your friends over and begin preparing—now you *have* to do it. That's what's special about the energy from your inspirations: It boosts you past the initial hurdle of starting.

My friend Tyrone had an idea when we were out clubbing. In his partying state, he had an awesome idea to create an app that allowed him to book tables at nightclubs in advance. In Asia, it's common to get tables in advance. If you have a table, you can get in without any hiccups; plus, you get to sit down and drink. But these tables were gated by people who decided the price based on how they were feeling. If the night was getting busy, the table prices just skyrocketed.

I laughed at Tyrone's idea and we kept drinking.

The next day we woke up in our suite, then sat at the kitchen table and complained about our hangover, like any self-respecting adult.

That was when I witnessed something ridiculous.

Tyrone received a message: "I have time, we could try make the app prototype in three months." Tyrone was confused.

Apparently, in his euphoric state the night before, he had sent a message to a bootstrapping developer he knew. Tyrone decided to meet with the developer and they went on to make the app.

I know you might be expecting to hear a story of an amazing application, but it didn't turn out that way. The app was made, but they ended up selling the prototype to a nightclub. They made some good money, and we went to the club again to celebrate.

Moral of the story? Don't drink. Actual moral of the story? *When you get an idea, force the next step.*

Why force yourself?

When you get a flash of inspiration, it makes you feel like you can do it. It feels like your goal is obtainable, even though every other day you feel like you shouldn't even try. Perhaps you were scared to do something before, but now? Now, you have that little extra kick to do it. Inspiration gets you over the initial hurdle, and then boosts you to the next step.

I have no doubt Tyrone would have never made that app if he hadn't messaged the developer. He may have convinced himself that his idea was stupid. He may have thought his friend would be busy. Or, most likely, he would have forgotten about it.

> *There are so many things we can tell ourselves to prevent us from achieving our goal. Flashes help you break that fear.*

Once you've gotten over the first hurdle, you are now tied to the idea. Have an incredible idea to start a business with a friend? Call him straight away and say, "Let's meet tomorrow. It's about a business idea I want to start." Your hesitations are gone. Your ability to reconsider the idea has vanished.

Remember, when distractions settle in that's when we lose our momentum. That's when we don't bother doing anything at all.

I've wasted many opportunities and I've probably lost many ideas simply because I didn't capitalize on that first moment. Here are a few simple things you can do to make sure you don't waste your flashes:

- Keep a book next to your bed because you never know what ideas may come at night.
- Set an alarm on your phone the moment your idea pops into your head; name it something memorable. Set a time when you know you will be free, so when the alarm rings it will remind you of your idea. Alternatively, you can use your phone's notes function to record key words, phrases, or core concepts that can re-trigger your ideas.
- Need to meet someone to get the ball rolling? Call them—now. You've discovered the treasure, so you got to let them know.

Find how your mind works and do what works for you. Just don't waste flashes. Flashes help you achieve your goal.

I still shake my head when I remember a friend of mine telling me he had the idea for PayPal or another person who told me she had the idea for Instagram. If you have an idea, and you execute on it instead of wasting a flash of inspiration, maybe it could be very successful!

The more committed you are to a specific idea, the more likely it is to start. Flashes of inspiration are rare and should not be wasted. You may never know when, or if, it will come again. Take the energy and run with it. That's how you achieve what you want.

9. YOU ARE ADDICTED TO MOTIVATION

Achievers don't need external motivation.

Motivation is a drug that makes you feel good. When you finish watching a motivational speech, you feel amazing. It empowers you to do something with your life. You go out and start your journey to success. This new energy can push you to achieve something amazing.

Or not.

Some people end up looking for the next motivational seminar or book they should get into. All they want is another hit of that "feel good" motivational drug.

Motivation becomes an endless cycle of feel good + no progress.

I understand how that endorphin rush you get when you read these inspirational books can get you hooked. I say this from experience because I have an extensive library of these books. However, without a plan to put what you've learned into action, all that knowledge is meaningless. You can endlessly read one book after another and they all say the exact same thing: You can do it!

All of a sudden we find ourselves meeting strangers and walking over fire because that somehow reflects our ability to be courageous and achieve success.

Motivation has a limit, and that limit is generally reached way before it becomes an addiction. If you go past that limit, you're basically mind-masturbating. Every time you feel like you don't have the energy, you read a motivating quote. When you don't know what to do, you watch a motivating speech or go to a new seminar.

Stop it.

This is a bad habit.

All motivation does is make you *feel* like you have done something, but in reality, you've done nothing. You've just found something that provides you with a fake sense of progress. I've done this before, many times.

And after all, here I am trying to motivate you by telling you motivation is a lie.

Motivation comes and goes. No matter your goal in life, if it's to become a marathon runner or a pro gamer, there are times you will feel like shit. There are times you will feel like you need a spark of energy.

When Stephen King tries to write a book, he sits there even when nothing comes to mind and writes until he reaches the goal he needs. He's willing to shovel through the crap. Do you think he reads some inspirational quote, and then an idea comes to him?

No way.

If you truly want something, you don't need motivation, you need to be able to grind through the crap to get to the gold. Did all these successful people just continually dose themselves up with motivation? Definitely not.

But wait, these Tony Robbins seminars are great! You know what, I think they are, too. And *Think and Grow Rich, Giant Within, Psycho-Cybernetics* are all amazing books I would still suggest to anyone pursuing success to read. But, after reading a few books, you will definitely see how they all share the same themes.

I'm shocked at how people jump from one inspirational seminar to the next and think they are progressing in their goals.

"Dude, you have to come."

"You aren't living if you haven't gone through this course."

It is as if everyone is missing out on something huge.

If you're truly motivated after coming out to one of these courses, then why are you going to another one? You want another hit of feel good. If you're really ready to go, you only need one good shot of motivation. The rest is just an addiction and a waste of time.

A friend of mine got caught up in this. She was so convinced that these conferences were making a big difference in her life that she would throw thousands of dollars at them. She would fly to different countries to try out different experiences. She met new people. She felt empowered. For years, she tried to convince me to go with her. When I told her it was a waste of time, she got defensive.

Now, it's years later and she hasn't done anything. She is still working the job she hated.

I was also addicted to motivation. But I wasn't addicted to conferences. Nope, I got my feel goods from books. Non-fiction/self-help top sellers? I've read them all. I even started reading obscure books. But the more you read, the more you distract yourself from actually *doing*. You can read. You can learn. But if you do not do, then that motivation is wasted.

It's like filling a car with gas, but you don't know where you plan to drive the car. Without a destination, it was better to just leave the car empty. At least you saved money on gas.

So, if you feel like you need some motivation, guess what? You don't.

You need to start actually dealing with shit. No life goal is going to be easy. Learning to walk is hard. Learning to talk is hard. Even learning how to type on a keyboard is hard. But you are forced to do that stuff if you want to get around and communicate. You are forced to weave through the crap, so you do it without a second thought.

I remember the first day of learning how to drive. I had no clue what the hell a clutch was let alone how to juggle between accelerating and changing gears. But now, I can karaoke to music, chew on beef jerky while driving— all at the same time!

Motivation is just a distraction. It's a way for you to delay dealing with the crap that's wrapped around you getting to your goal. So, stop motivational masturbating. Go deal with the shit that comes with mastering or achieving your goals.

You might hate having to deal with life's challenges. Maybe you hate thinking about what you need to do to achieve your goals. You have to sign up to a class? *Great, this is going to be boring.* You have to meet more people? *Urgh – meeting more strangers!*

But you got to do it.

No one achieved anything sitting and listening to motivational porn.
Figure out where the car needs to go, then fill it up with gas.

10. YOU SAY YOU DON'T HAVE ENOUGH TIME

"I don't have enough time."

This is by far the most common excuse anyone can make. It was just the other day that I walked past a colleague who saw me typing on my laptop. She asked what I was doing. I told her I was writing a book.

Her response was, "You can only do that because you have the time."

I was tempted to tell her that she has the time, too, since when she was talking to me, she was browsing through her social media.

But I didn't, as I realize that she might get defensive.

If you genuinely think you don't have *time* to achieve things, then you won't achieve what you want. It's as simple as that. No time means you are admitting you can't do it. Story ends.

But what the fuck would I know, right?

A friend once told me that anyone can make the time if they want something enough. At first, I thought, *what an asshole*. It sounded like he was telling me how to run my life. *As if I wasn't trying my best already.* I immediately went on the defensive.

"I'm doing whatever I can, man, I just don't have time."

He then told me to look at the 168-hour rule. Why 168 hours? It's because that's the total number of hours we're allotted in any given week.

The rule is simple: Break down your week by hours to find how many real hours you have left. Ten hours for work, six days a week make for sixty hours a week. Two hours a day for eating. I added everything up. No matter how hard I tried to prove my excuse of no time, I still had at least fifteen hours a week left over.

It was impossible to say I didn't have time.

In my head, all I could say was, *Where the fuck did my time go?*

But I still fought him on it. "Nah, there must be a mistake."

He shrugged it off with a *whatever* and we ended up talking about other random things. When I went home that day, I realized the "rule" had left an impression with me.

What *was* consuming my time?

I started being more conscious about what I was doing and for how long. I was scrolling on social media. I was reading news headlines, and then googling whatever I could find. I was sitting at the computer, mindlessly thinking of what to do next.

I had time. I was just wasting it. And if you waste time, you won't achieve anything.

There are people who will argue that they still can't find the time. They will tell you that their schedule is so packed that 168 hours isn't even enough! If that's truly the case, then you *must* cut out something to free up some time. Saying you don't have the time to work on your goals, and at the same time saying it's impossible to find the time means you simply can't work on your goals. The end.

Either accept that or cut the bullshit.

For me, it was not having the time to exercise. I continually made the excuse that my day was always jammed packed. So, I had to make a choice: Cut the time I was sleeping or simply concede that I had no time to exercise. I took thirty minutes from my sleep to jog in the morning.

Was it hard to wake up? Sure was. But I got used to it.

Always ask yourself what is worth cutting. What will allow you to have time to achieve what you want.

Now I know a lot of people won't want to cut their sleep. Paul, a program developer, told me he preferred to program at night. He liked the quietness and he was just more productive when it was eerily silent. Although he was required to work the usual hours of the day, he told his boss his preference and he was able to work at night instead. This gave him far more productive hours at work.

However, not everyone has this luxury. Doctors and dentists can't just work at night. Banks and shops are open during normal shopping hours and can't just change their open times.

But the point here is that Paul figured out his most efficient time.

So, find yours. Dedicate that time to your goal. Move your schedule so that the most efficient time is allocated to what deserves it. Not to video games or watching TV shows, but your actual goals.

And if you're one of those people who fight back and say it's still not possible, then maybe it's time to start questioning how much you really want to achieve your goal. Do you want it or not?

I have often been asked where I find the time to do other things. My friend on Facebook messaged me after I posted about a game I developed in my spare time. Their message said, "You have a lot of time on your hands." Yet, I see his videos and stories, his partying, drinking, and gaming. He doesn't have any perception of his own time, and when he sees other people do actual shit, he simply thinks other people just have more time than him. Fuck that.

Time is your most valuable resource. It is finite for everyone.

When my colleague asked me what I was doing, I said I was writing my book on my lunch break. I made time. I found moments in my life that I could use to achieve what I wanted. When I was headed to a party with a friend, the taxi ride was going to be an hour. What was he doing? Studying Mandarin on his palm cards.

You find little breaks of time to work on your goals. It may seem impossible or stupid, but you have to do it.

You have to fight for your time. You have to squeeze out any free moment you can. I may only get to write a single sentence or learn one new word, but that's one step in the right direction.

Time can be made if you really set your mind to it; otherwise, you apparently don't give a fuck about your goal. If you did, you wouldn't make an excuse. You really do have time.

If you still think you don't have the time, then just give up; you will never achieve what you want.

11. YOU SPEND TOO LONG IN THE DOWNSWINGS

When I broke up with my first girlfriend I was shattered. I spent months doing absolutely nothing. There were times I lay in my bed just staring at the ceiling. I have no idea what I was thinking; I just sat around and moped. I remember sitting in a park and crying.

It was some sad shit if I do say so myself. But was I feeling sorry for myself? No, I was just wasting time.

Months later, she had moved on and dated my friend. I let that get to me and I just fell into a deeper hole. I was shattered and felt like doing nothing at all. I let it get the best of me, and because of that, I missed many amazing opportunities and scared away friends.

You may go through something similar, and the reason you don't achieve shit during that time is because you spend too long in the down period of your life.

Last year, I made a promising investment in a Vietnamese company, a manufacturer for farming equipment. I had done my due diligence and met with the business owners.

For a few months things were going very well, but then one of the owners decided to shaft his business partner and I.

He saw how profitable the business was and decided to open a shop of his own. He then funneled our clients to his own store and put the business into liquidation.

I was fueled with anger, but had no idea how to fix it. I had no clue what I could really do, and after talking to lawyers and friends, all the signs pointed to giving up.

I spent months trying to figure out how to get my revenge. I spent money and time hatching a plan. I wasted mental space and resources. I could have used that time to plan my next venture or investment. I spent too long in the downswing—and achieved absolutely nothing.

It's not uncommon to see people completely broken after a traumatic event. It's not wrong to feel sad or upset. But the world keeps moving. And while you're standing still, it will leave you behind. The longer the world spins without you, the more you will have to play catch up.

How on earth do you plan to achieve the stuff you want, when all you are doing is spinning your wheels in the muck? You must minimize the time you are down.

I have a friend, Tony, who was in a down period once and it was absolutely upsetting to see.

He had started a small media company during the dotcom boom. He had investors who helped him financially and supported his company. Things were on the rise. He was going to be successful.

I remember one particular party where I learned that champagne bottles would be sliced open with a credit card. At that party one of the investors had drank a little too much and let slip that he couldn't wait to "sell the company."

Tony had no idea what he meant and pretty much stopped drinking the whole night. The next day, he found out the investors planned to sell his company. They were in the right, too, so he couldn't do anything about it. The worst part was Tony wouldn't end up with much after the company was sold. His shares were diluted as the company grew and he had barely anything left.

He became a walking zombie after learning all this.

But his ability to grow a successful company had built his reputation. People knew him and wanted him to join their firms. One offer was an amazing opportunity in Melbourne. He was to become a CEO of a data analytic company. Another offer was to join a growing consulting firm for entrepreneurs. People wanted him and I was jealous!

But he was in deep, moping around. He was in love with the company he had built and wanted it back. He glossed over the offers and kept thinking of what he had lost. He was stuck in an endless cycle of negative thinking. One time he desperately called the company to let him buy it back. He sounded like a dog begging for food. They said no.

Over time, he turned to drinking and smoking. Soon it went to partying and drugs. In the background, he let the offers die. His reputation faded away, and instead of becoming a legend, he became a fucking nobody.

He missed a lot of opportunities for sure. For example, the data company was a huge success because it latched onto the concept of artificial intelligence.

Do not be Tony.

You will miss shit you may never have a chance at again.

The world does not give a fuck about you.

If you break up in a relationship there is nothing wrong with grieving. If you lose money in a deal, then I'd be surprised if you didn't feel upset. But you want to achieve, right? You want to hit your goals, right?

So, you need to minimize the down times.

Life *will* have ups and downs. Even the highest achievers I know have downswings. But it's *how long* they spend in those downswings that matters the most. The difference between these non-achievers and people who actually get shit done is how long they spend at the bottom.

Julian was similar to Tony even though he didn't run a successful company. However, he had an uncanny way of getting over things very quickly. At first, I thought he was cold. When his girlfriend dumped him, in the next few days he seemed happy. Maybe he was keeping up a front, but it was definitely shocking to see him carry on with life as if nothing had happened.

But the part I remember most was when he lost his job. For a few days he was upset. We hung out a bit later and he told me he was already looking for jobs. I was shocked. My instinct was to tell him it was okay to grieve, but he didn't even need it. He just got the fuck up and looked for the next thing.

Where is he now? He's a management consultant in a top-tier firm. He didn't let shit faze him.

Someone told me to "keep your chin up" when I had broken up with my girlfriend. I thought it was just some poor attempt to make me feel better.

But it wasn't. Really, you *should* keep your chin up. When shit happens, the person who succeeds is the one who gets up and does something about it. If there's an earthquake, the people we look to are the ones who are calm and know what to do.

When I was sad, I always looked down. I refused to go out. I missed shit that was around me. I missed the friends that were supportive. I missed the "next thing" to work on. The longer I spent being sad or angry, the more I failed to see the things around me.

That's how brutal the world is. It will not wait for you. The people around you, as much as they may care, will not give any fucks about you the longer you stand still doing nothing. Moral of the story: Keep moving. Chin up or let the world leave you behind.

12. YOU CONCENTRATE ON THINGS OUT OF YOUR CONTROL

It is very easy to concentrate on the things you can't control. Take, for example, the coronavirus. When the pandemic started in my city, jobs were lost, relationships became strained, and the lingering uncertainty felt like shit. You had no clue what to do, who had the virus, and what was going to happen.

Since we have a tendency to concentrate on what we can't control, I started to think of what would happen to my relationships and my finances. *Would I be kicked out of my property if I can't afford the rent? Will I never be able to work again?*

This kind of thinking can be a never-ending cycle.

You won't achieve shit if you let events outside your control dictate what you do.

Instead of worrying about my rent, I should have taken stock of my current financial situation. Instead of crying about any lack of work, I could have looked at my own skill sets to find a way to make money or look for another job.

I was stuck thinking about things I couldn't control. It is so tempting, and so easy, to get lost in it. You think of the problems and factors you have absolutely no influence over and the result is *doing* nothing.

I have seen countless business meetings go nowhere just because no one looks at what is controllable. You can't control how your competitor responds. You can't control Mother Nature, tsunamis, earthquakes—or a virus. You can work on *how* you respond to such events. You can work on your next move.

You can look at what you have and plan your next attack. If your goals are failing, you must find out what you *can* control to achieve it. The factors you can't? Just accept them and move on.

One time, a friend had an interview and a truck drove by, splashing dirty water on his suit. He panicked. He complained and whined. He spent the last half hour before his interview building up anger about his soiled suit. He was flustered and still mad when he met the interviewer.

He didn't get the job.

When he complained to a bunch of friends the next day, I noticed he didn't look at things he could have controlled. Instead, he fixated on things completely out of control. He got angry about the *already* dirty suit. He got angry at the truck driver, *who was already driving away.* He got upset at fate. He didn't look at solutions. Why not make up a funny story about the suit? Why not go buy a new suit? Why not have a good laugh instead of just getting angry?

You must work with what you can control so you can always move forward toward your goals.

How you respond may be what decides if you can achieve something you want. What will you do—or could you do—if your plan fucks up?

Our goals will not always work out as we had planned. So, you need to adapt; you need to work with what you have. You will not achieve what you want if you don't seek solutions to whatever arises. There is no universal solution for any single problem. What will work for you might not work for others. The resources you have may not be available to others.

The only way to solve obstacles you will inevitably come across is to work on what you can control. If you're about to get married and it starts raining, why complain? Get everyone inside, find a new location, or delay the event.

If you screw up a performance because some kid was crying in the audience, don't blame the kid.

What can you actually control?

If you focus on what you can't control, you give energy and attention to shit that has already happened and doesn't matter now.

There are many people who won't achieve anything simply because they focus on things that are uncontrollable. In any situation, you can influence the outcome, but you can never control it.

I remember overhearing two staff members talking about how people were getting laid off. They started to worry about what would happen to them. *What if I get fired? Do I need to find a new job? Will I be okay?* One got so worked up about it that she was in tears. She looked fragile and worried. It affected her mental state and she could barely do any work for the rest of the day. But her fears were all about situations that hadn't even happened.

One did get fired eventually, and you can guess which one. She didn't work on changing the outcome, on what she could have controlled. Instead of waiting for doom, she could have showed her energy at work. She could have asked what other jobs she could do. There were so many roads to take, but she took the one that didn't even exist. She ended up creating the scenario she feared most.

There is an amazing feeling that comes when you influence outcomes by working on things you can control. It empowers you to change other things in your life. Your effort and energy don't go to waste because you can now concentrate on the things that actually matter. Crazily, you will start to forget the things you can't control.

You will know that variables do exist when you try to achieve something, and this gives you greater confidence even when you fail. You can reflect on things that will genuinely help you achieve what you want. You pick yourself up and do it again. You fine-tune the things you can change.

So, leave behind the things you can't control and focus on what you can. Let others waste their time. Don't get caught up in their shit and don't let shit consume your head. Any time you feel like things aren't working your way, take a deep breath.

What can you control?

What factors are out of your control? Wipe them out. Change what you can. No journey will be easy and wasting time on things you can't change, won't help.

In order for you to obtain your goals, you must focus
solely on factors you can influence.

13. YOU DON'T KNOW THE SECRET TO MOTIVATION

What does it mean to believe? Belief may be the only thing you have left when everything goes to shit and the world tells you your project is not worth it.

People accuse you of wasting your time. You have no money left and have been scraping by on a paltry part-time job. If nothing goes to plan, what do you have left?

Belief.

You need to believe you will achieve it. Yes, it sounds like some mumbo jumbo bullshit, but if you don't believe you can get whatever it is you want—when shit hits you in the face—you will call it quits. If you call it quits, you won't achieve your goals.

There are countless authors who strive to get their book published, and even when they are rejected and are told it will fail, they still try to publish it. Why? Because they believe in their book.

How does an entrepreneur stand in front of multiple venture capitalists, each one rejecting her and her idea? Because she believes in her product.

Belief is the one thing that will keep you motivated.

I was told to stop thinking of opening my own medical practice. I was convinced to quit. I needed money to start my idea, but no one would even spare me the time of day. Every time I tried to convince investors that I could do it, they all said it wasn't possible. After all, what does a fresh graduate know?

No luck.

I *did* think of giving up. It's very easy to finally say, *That's it. Why bother going on? It's clear this won't work.*

You start to convince yourself that everyone else is right.

You lose belief.

You quit.

But I didn't stop, and I was lucky I didn't.

I remember waiting outside the meeting room where I would speak to investors. I told myself this was going to be the last shot I take. As the receptionist told me to come in, I realized this was an "all in" move. After this, I would go work for someone else, save enough money, and do it myself.

The pitch went by so quickly.

I told the investors of my plan and the trickle of belief I had left kept me going. Things just started flowing, and by the end of my presentation, an investor told me to stop.

"Let's do it, I believe in you."

Ironic, isn't it? I had almost quit believing in myself. I signed the papers the following week and got the money to move forward.

I always wondered: If I had given up before this last-ditch effort, what would have happened? I'm fortunate to never know, but if I didn't believe in myself the other times I was rejected, it would have ended right there and then.

So, what really is the secret to motivation?

It is starting with something you believe in. If you believe in it, nothing will stop you.

When my friend lost her job, she had an unwavering belief that she could become a doctor. She wanted to go back to study medicine, even with all the years it entailed.

When she asked me what my opinion was, I thought she was joking. It was a ridiculous goal. Bar all the logistics aside, it would be a grueling path. She would have to manage studies, a mortgage, and work a job on the side.

But last year she graduated. I was there and watched her celebrate her achievement. *She actually fucking did it*, I thought.

When she was around all her friends and family, she was told to give a little speech. She told us that when she was working overtime or night shifts, she almost gave up. When a patient told her to fuck off because she was trying to give them medication, she went home in tears.

But she believed in herself. She kept going.

No matter what the world throws in your face, you hold onto that belief. That is what keeps you going.

Some people will tell others their beliefs are wrong. Honestly, who cares what another person's beliefs are? Do you care?

If others believe in their pyramid scheme, so be it. As long as it doesn't affect you, you really shouldn't give a shit. If they believe in their product so much, the more you fight them, the more likely they will defend themselves. Don't waste time on the beliefs of others.

Worry about your own belief because that is all that matters.

Your beliefs will always be challenged. But think of those challenges as tests to see how much you want something. If one person is able to convince you that you can't obtain what you want, then clearly you don't deserve it.

If multiple people can change your mind, well, just give up. These attempts to foil your beliefs may come from family, friends, or even strangers. No matter how it comes to you, you will be challenged. The more challengers, the harder it gets.

You need conviction to stand your ground to achieve what you want. Actors do it. Comedians do it. MBA students do it. Everyone who succeeds does it and has done it. How well you stand up for your beliefs matters.

Whether your belief is in your project, yourself, or the idea you want to try, you must believe in it.

Belief will be the only thing that supports you when shit hits the fan—and shit *will* hit the fan.

Don't think that when you are challenged you must concede and admit you are wrong. Those challenges are a test—to truly see how much you believe in yourself and your idea/dream/goal.

At the root of achievement is belief.

PART II

YOUR GOALS

Your goals are your priority.
Make a plan. Execute it.

14. YOU AREN'T REAL
WITH YOUR GOALS

Do you want money? Is it for expensive things? Or perhaps you want to raise a family. Maybe you just want to be famous on social media. Be honest. Be really honest. There's nothing wrong with wanting money. There's nothing wrong with vanity. There's nothing wrong with simply wanting to raise a family.

If that is truly what you want, then you should go for it.

But.

If you can't be true to yourself, you won't achieve it. You must at least have a *real* goal in mind. Not a goal you read in a book or a goal your friends told you about, but a goal that genuinely reflects what *you* want.

I was at a dinner once and I told friends about my current goal. I wanted a specific apartment. It wasn't just a standard house; it was one of those penthouses with a view that you could show off. Even I admit it was ridiculously vain.

The moment I said it, people were judging. There was an awkward shift among those seated at the table. Eyes opened wide in disbelief. My friend, who sat next to me, was confused but decided to break the silence, saying, "That's really materialistic."

And it really was.

So what? There will always be people who think your goal is stupid or selfish. And there will be others with the exact same goal.

I once met a man who didn't have a family. He was rich as fuck. He had a small plane and a boat he rarely used. I really loved his selection of cars and I'm sure he loved showing them to me. Did he want more money? Yes. He would party with friends, go home and continue making more money. The guy was greedy as fuck! Did people judge him? 100%. More cars? More money? He loved it.

Was he happy? *Yes.* He was then, and still is. I'm certain he has added more cars to his garage by now. Probably another boat as well.

In a different city, I know a photographer who loves to travel. He can't afford expensive flights and works day-by-day to make enough to travel regularly. I met him by pure luck as he was waiting tables in Canada. He travels for experiences and takes photos of places you and I never get to see. Some of those areas are barren, but I must say he sure convinced me that deserts are beautiful. Do I plan to visit those places? Hell no!

He lives for the moments. He lives to see unique things in life. He gives zero fucks about money. Is he happy? *Yes.*

Would these two people talk to each other if they crossed paths? Definitely not. One is in a suit most of the time, the other is dressed like he doesn't have a home (he actually doesn't). But they have one thing in common: *They are happy.*

They know what they want. They based their direction in life on just that. When you stop caring about what other people think of your life goals, you can move in the right direction.

Knowing what makes you tick will help you achieve your goal.

You need to find what really sets you off. What sets a fire inside you? If you want a private jet, then so be it. Go for it. Who cares if it's materialistic? Why change your goals because of what others tell you?

When you become really honest in what you want, things will start to align. It gives you a reason to go to work. It will consume your free time and be what you think about before you fall to sleep. Things are aligned in one direction, and that's toward achieving your goal.

This isn't about passion.

This is about what will drive you to do your very best. What will push you on the days you feel like doing absolutely nothing? Find what makes you tick and remind yourself of it.

In the book, *The Top Five Regrets of the Dying*, the greatest regret people have on their deathbed is "I wish I'd had the courage to live a life true to myself, not the life others expected of me."

Sometimes your goal isn't really yours. We all know someone who is living someone else's dream. Perhaps it's from their parents, their friends, or their loved ones. Someone has convinced them what they are doing is wrong. Although it is possible to finish goals you haven't made for yourself, doing so is a lot harder. You will have less drive. You are less likely to achieve it.

So, be honest. You cannot afford to base your reason to do something based on what other people tell you. You won't know straight away, but that's why you start.

When you do anything, your own personal reason is the most important. You know when someone says "your heart isn't in it"? It's because it probably isn't. If you don't want to give to charity, then don't. If you want to help people who are homeless, then do it. If you want fame, *go for it.*

You aren't being greedy. You aren't being too selfish. You are making one person happy in this world—you. When you die, and yes, we all die, you will die pursuing what you wanted.

You don't have time to be unhappy doing something you don't like. You do have time to do things you want from this world. So, when you set yourself out to make a goal yours, be honest with what you value. Memories? Moments? Likes on your Instagram? It doesn't matter what it is! Base yourself on it!

Whatever the fuck you want, be proud, say it out loud.

So, make your move. Your internal compass will lead you to different places. Sometimes you aren't sure, sometimes you feel the fear set in, but you must keep moving. It will direct you to where you need to go. The people, the places, and the moments you make will be based on your reason.

Even if you move to toward something and you don't like it, at least you know where not to go next time. Moving is a lot better than standing still. Be real—or you ain't going to achieve shit.

15. YOU ARE NEGOTIABLE WITH YOUR GOALS

It's late at night and someone calls you. You're learning to play piano for the first time. It's something you've always wanted to master but never had the time to finish. You stop playing the piece of music and you pick up your phone. Your friend asks you to go out for a drink. It's a bit unexpected but seeing your friends is part of your priorities, too, right?

You get changed and head out. Dust builds on the piano. You come home drunk and spend tomorrow recovering. You think to yourself, *Why the fuck did I go out last night?*

We make plans.

I, for one, love making New Year's Resolution plans. Just before the year ticks over I formulate a juicy plan about how I'm going to achieve something. This plan is beautiful because it accommodates for everything. It's a fucking masterpiece. Yet even after making this state-of-the-art plan, I have failed year after year.

One year I planned to be fluent in Korean. That took me nowhere. The moment a friend asked me to play computer games or to go out and grab a drink, I went. I think of reasons why it's better to *not* work on my goals. I disregard the plan I made. The schedules I made to learn and study Korean became so low priority that I might as well have not made the plan at all.

It was the "making" of the plan that felt good. That felt like progress to me. But a plan is not enough. If you create one, you must be committed to doing it.

You must set some time aside to do what you want. That time should be 100% dedicated to the goal. Distractions should be removed. Anything that can remotely affect your concentration must be completely erased. If it isn't, why the fuck did you set it up in the first place? I'm not saying cancel emergency calls. If my parents called to say something was wrong or a close friend is about to die, holy shit, I'd want to know as soon as possible. But if it's something less than life-or-death, you really need to think about it. Can it wait? Most things can. In all my years, I have never had that "emergency" call, so now I just shut my phone off all together.

One time, I remember working on some code for a video game due for release in a few weeks. While I was smashing my head on the keyboard, I received a call from a friend. There was a big party in town and my friend told me he could get me in. It wasn't a big famous celebrity party, but it seemed to be one I apparently "should not miss."

I wasted two hours deciding if I should go. Maybe I could go for an hour, then come back. I put on a jacket. Minutes later, I took off the jacket and decided not to go. The game was more important to me.

By spending that additional time coding, my company could create a viral GIF on Reddit. Had I gone to the party, I'm sure I would have met some cool people. But in the end, you make a choice. You can't be everywhere all the time.

You will have to miss some engagements. You will miss some important people and meetings. You just need to make sure you prioritize what is most important to you.

When I was young, I was forced to do Taekwondo. Yes, forced. My parents dropped me off at the gym and I had to go. My God, was I a cry baby. I didn't like it at first. In fact, through the first four full belts I tried to actually avoid going by pretending I was sick. One day I even pretended I had a terrible sprain and my leg was broken. It didn't work.

Eventually the lessons wore on me, but more importantly, I actually got good at Taekwondo! My parents made it non-negotiable and, in the end, I got a black belt. Good? Bad? Doesn't matter. I get to strut around to my friends that I'm a black belt.

Point is, if you ever had lessons in music or sports, you had a set amount of time with the instructor. You couldn't do anything else. You sat there, listened, and did it. You may have even hated it. But you still improved because there was nothing else you could really do *but* improve.

You had to show up and dedicate yourself for a whole lesson. Sounds horrible, hey? But dammit, it worked.

So, when you set a portion of your day to your goal, you make sure it can't be touched.

No one touches your goal time. This is the time you set
yourself to fucking achieve.

We spend a lot of time making a plan for our goals. If you spend that long making a plan, why would you allow something to get in the way? If you don't plan to stick to it, just tear it up and hope one day you can commit to it.

So, when you are being asked to negotiate with your goals—maybe a friend or family member that needs your time—the answer is: *no.*

Your goals are non-negotiable.

16. YOU DON'T SET REAL DEADLINES

I have always wondered why, in college, I could finish an essay that I had no interest in, but when I wanted to publish a book, I couldn't even get the first sentence written.

The difference? I had a teacher who would fail me for not completing the essay. If I didn't finish it, she would tell my parents. My parents would probably proceed to beat me or confiscate my Super Nintendo. I didn't care about the beating, but my Super Nintendo? That possessed the power of Mario Kart and Bomberman.

You cannot lose that.

So, I finished the damn essay. It had a deadline with consequence.

We don't get things done because we stop setting deadlines.

This book is about achievement, and people who actually achieve something have a deadline. If you don't set a deadline, you would have an infinite amount of time to finish something. That would mean you could take your damn sweet time. You could have days to tell yourself, *You know what? Let's do it tomorrow.* Other days you could work a little bit on your goals, but then your friend tells you there's a new pop up organic-no-meat-BPA-free burger joint and you decide to go.

Without deadlines, whatever you want to achieve is left on the backburner over and over again.

So, what happens if your friend calls you about this amazing restaurant, but you look on your calendar and realize that your manuscript for your editor is due tomorrow? Or you have to submit your game design to a game development company? You will tell your friend, no. You will say *what a shame I'm going to miss out on this burger joint* and you will work on your goal. You say no because there's something that's more important. Its importance came because you gave it a deadline.

However, a deadline alone is not enough.

Anyone can just set a random date. If I had a dollar for every time I set a random date to get something done, such as *next week, tomorrow or next year,* I would have enough money to open a burger joint. This type of procrastination isn't uncommon. You could ask a friend when they would get something done and very rarely are they able to give you a specific date.

My personal adventure into deadlines was because of something very vain. I have always wanted six-pack abs. After seeing *Captain America and Fight Club*, I just felt that was what I needed. Like anyone starting out with exercising, I did the smallest amount possible. I YouTube'd eight-minute abs. I did it on and off for a year and didn't get any results. I was tired of it. I decided to do something different. I called a photographer and set up a topless photography shoot.

What was I thinking, right?

I figured since my goal was vain, it would make sense I would feel very awkward if I looked pudgy for a photo shoot. I paid *in advance* for the photo shoot and scheduled it ten weeks ahead.

Things change once you have a clear deadline. Losing weight doesn't happen overnight, and the bigger your goal, the more you start to realize it will take time. You then know you can't procrastinate. You can't just cram it at the very end. You have to start *now.*

That's what I did.

I changed my diet and became more disciplined in my exercising. By the 10-week mark, I didn't have ripped abs, but they were almost visible. I was proud to achieve what I set out to do. Since then, I have set deadlines with consequences.

Becoming accountable for your goal is important.

A deadline is not enough without some form of accountability. Are you certain you will get there? If you have any doubt, tell someone who is extremely close to you or even make a punishment for not getting there.

A friend of mine told me she would save $1000 in three months because she had a bad spending habit. Otherwise, any money and anything she bought during those three months she would donate to charity.

Another colleague of mine said if he didn't run a marathon in six months, he would give me his signed jersey from Michael Jordan. He ran it in two months. Yes, I was tempted to make him go out and eat fatty foods so he wouldn't run it. I'm a horrible friend!

These deadlines may sound silly at first, but they can be powerful driving forces.

With a deadline in place you can see how long you have and what you have to do. You don't have to do anything extreme; just make yourself accountable.

So, when you're ready to set your goals, make sure that they're specific and have a deadline because *you don't have forever.*

Give yourself a deadline with consequences.

Don't give power to distractions and things that prevent you from achieving what you want. The larger the goal, the earlier you have to start putting effort toward achieving it.

No goal is complete without a finish line.

17. YOU CREATE DISTRACTIONS

As I type this line, I'm so tempted to look at my phone. My phone is flickering, and I want to see who has messaged me. I'm not immune to distractions, no one really is. A phone that lights up when sitting between two people means someone is going to look at it.

My phone is there because I put it there. I am responsible for the distraction. In order to achieve, you've got to say *fuck you, distraction!* and not allow it to even be in the room with you.

Some days, I disconnect the Wi-Fi because the Internet is distracting me. Other days, I put the phone on silent and put it in another room. Any distraction that is near you or interrupts you as you work on your goals is *your responsibility.*

Can't get shit done because you are distracted? It's *your fault.*

It's impossible to achieve your goal if you have distractions. If you work better in a café, then do so. If you work better at home, stay home. *These are choices you get to make.* I have heard countless friends tell me that they can't get anything done because they are at home. *So, why don't you just leave home?*

I am surprised how people can rationalize the distractions they feel they must deal with.

A friend of mine who was trying to study the GMAT (an exam to get into graduate school) had her phone right next to her all the time. The moment it flashed, she would pick it up and looked to see who it was. Even during timed exam sessions, it was always next to her.

When she asked me ways for her to improve her concentration, I asked her if her phone was *that* important. At first, she defended how much she needed it in case the phone rang, but all that ever came were messages from friends about random things. No excuse worked. In the end, she agreed she needed to stop checking her phone and ended with a 99 percentile GMAT score.

Her issue was never about the phone though because some people can work with a phone right in front of them. Heck, some can work with their social media flashing in their face. However, if it puts you in a different mindset or distracts you from working on achieving your goal, it's got to go.

All goals require your complete attention. Why work on a goal if you can't do that? Distractions keep you from getting into and maintaining the rhythm of what you are working on. Some of my most productive work occurs because I have nothing else to do *but* work.

Have you ever had an idea that you wanted to work on but the moment your phone rings, you forget everything you were doing? It's the worst feeling. It could take ages for you to get back into it. I've been guilty of wasting hours because of a simple distraction: mobile phone games.

But in today's world, stimulation is the norm. There are seemingly unlimited distractions and our attention spans are getting shorter. No wonder we don't achieve shit!

You could be sitting on a million-dollar idea, a life-changing experience, or meeting the love your life, but because of that damn email, you missed out. Truth: If distractions take all your attention, your goals get none. It's as simple as that.

I once decided to track how many hours I consumed using apps that I deemed were distractions: Web browsing, social media, video games, and Netflix. After a week, I thought I had really minimized my distractions.

My time was 15 hours and 23 minutes. That's an average of two hours a day. I was disgusted. So, even when I was trying, I still let these programs distract me and prevent me from achieving my goals.

Another distraction and problem we face in achieving our goals is running on other people's time. Damien, a consultant I knew, was stuck to his device. When he was trying to start his own business, his phone always had a large number of unread emails. It looked like an endless parade of notifications. His phone seeped into every part of his life, even his exercise. While jogging, he was on his phone. In between sets at the gym, he was checking his phone. One set—check; another set—check. Every set was done poorly. Even when he had a personal trainer, he looked at his phone. He ended up quitting the gym, saying it wasn't getting him anywhere.

Damien was running on other people's schedules.

Later, instead of checking his emails incessantly, he scheduled certain times to complete this task.

What happened with his clients?

Nothing. Everything was the same.

But his life? It improved drastically. He could spend more time with his wife and kids and work more on his health.

If someone sends you a message and you instantly reply, you are working on their time. You are letting someone else dictate what you are doing. How do you plan to achieve anything if you operate on another person's clock?

A few years ago, I was in a room with friends, discussing business ideas. We threw the craziest ideas at each other. One of my favorites was called "the Uber for packages"—but by plane.

People have limitations when they travel, but some travelers don't use their carry limits, so we thought it would be cool to have people bring parcels into other countries for you. But then, we realized one problem: If someone put something dodgy in the parcels, the passenger would have no clue. The idea was stupid. We threw it out.

But at some point, we had good ideas and people began texting other people about them. And soon, all conversation stopped. Everyone was glued to their phone, distracted and no longer discussing ideas with those present. All the energy we had created together was going into their phones. And then … we just let the ideas die away.

I'll never know if one of those ideas would have made us millions.

Don't let distractions prevent you from achieving what you want.

Cut them out of your life so you can concentrate on building a business, learning a new language or becoming a tennis star. Don't let small things like a flashing light on your phone or an email alert stop you from actually *doing* and achieving. Insignificant distractions can make a huge impact on the time you dedicate to your goals.

Turn the phone off.

Cut the distractions.

Don't run on other people's time.

18. YOU DON'T MAKE GOALS CHALLENGING

It's very tempting to work on the *easy* things. And why not? When things are easy, it's fun. Too bad easy doesn't help you move toward your goals.

Imagine if I told you to study the same Spanish language cards over and over again. If you aren't fluent in Spanish, it would be difficult at first, but each day you would improve in learning those same words. But what happens if that was all you did? What if the cards never changed or got more difficult? You'd become a master of the particular words you learned, but you wouldn't be fluent in Spanish. You'd hit a plateau due to your limited learning and make no further progress.

Learning the same things over and over again won't help you get anywhere. To achieve your goals, you must *challenge yourself*.

Playing a new piano piece? Make sure it contains challenges that allow you to learn something new. Learning a new word? Why not make it a sentence instead? Challenge yourself just a little bit more. If you don't, you will end up failing to achieve your goals because limited efforts will never get you where you need to go.

I learned from a friend, who was struggling to improve his Vietnamese, about why it is important to set difficult goals. He was going to be in charge of a factory in Vietnam and he needed to improve his Vietnamese in a hurry. So, every day, he increased the difficulty of his learning. He had a saying, "If I'm feeling comfortable, then I should be worried." And, the moment things got easy, he made things harder, ratcheting up the difficulty.

Similar to body builders who are working on building muscle: If you don't increase either the amount of reps or the weight you're lifting, your muscle shrinks.

You must keep challenging yourself and continually working on your discipline. If you set a goal that is too easy, you simply won't do it. Why would you do something you already know you can do?

One day at a party, a friend of mine, Tony, started to tell a group of us about his journey in poker. Recently, he had been very successful and wanted to share his winning formula.

"I started actually doing the hard shit," he told us. We all laughed and raised our glasses.

But what he said resonated with me. When I finally wanted some more sober poker tips, he revealed to me what he meant: He started playing against more challenging players.

Normally, he would play against the same people. Although he was winning, every time he played against other players or in a tournament with strangers, he would lose spectacularly. He finally had enough.

By playing against new people, he started losing, but he was able to learn more. "I realized that I had gotten used to how the regulars play. I wasn't improving my game. I was no longer learning."

From then on (at least up until now), he has been on a very good run. Challenges improve you. You don't learn anything sitting at the same table.

Some of the biggest achievements in your life will be remembered because they were challenging. A marathon, achieving blackbelt in Taekwondo, or winning a poker tournament: These are monumental goals. To achieve this level of achievement, you need to continually challenge yourself.

But a challenging goal does not mean an impossible goal.

Take for example, the iconic Dragon's Back hike in Hong Kong. It features a high and seemingly insurmountable peak. And yet, I could see the top. Impossible? It felt like it at first, but I could see where I needed to go and the trail before me that would get me there. Just seeing the peak of that mountain kept me going—kept me motivated.

So, I started climbing. Sure enough, the more I climbed, the closer the peak got. Was it challenging? Is altitude sickness a thing?

Yes and yes. However, when I reached the top, what had seemed impossible was suddenly possible.

When you set a challenging goal, you don't make it impossible. You make it within the realms of possibility.

Even when I made my first YouTube video I felt a sense of accomplishment. I look back at how I taught myself editing, watched endless guides on YouTube, and set up the green screen. Seeing it all tied together into a video gave me a sense that I could do something that I felt I couldn't. Setting and completing challenging goals is a remarkable feeling.

Challenging does not mean impossible; it just means it's really damn hard.

The more challenging the goal, the more satisfaction you will get from reaching it. No one can take that away from you. You will find that these monumental goals tend to be the ones you want to share. You will look forward to others asking you about it. You will have a damn epic story to tell. You accomplished it, so why not?

Challenges drives us. It gives us energy and excitement. It improves us. Most important, it will help you achieve your goals.

19. YOU DON'T TRACK YOUR PROGRESS

Imagine you're digging a tunnel. When you start digging, you can see how much dirt you were shoveling aside. As you shovel, you can see the dirt that's being thrown away. You can see the tunnel slowly starting to form. This gives you an incredible feeling, you feel like you can do anything.

But the more and more you dig, the deeper the tunnel gets. As you get further into the tunnel, it gets a lot harder to figure out how far you've come and how far you've got left to dig. That's normal, but sooner or later you feel like you aren't getting anywhere, so you give up. You throw the shovel away. You don't achieve a completed tunnel. Instead, all you have is just a giant pile of dirt.

That's what it is like to *not* track progression.

Quantify the goal as much as you can. Writing a book? Count how many words you're writing every day. Losing weight? Keep track of the weight and what your final weight will be. Saving money? Be clear about how much you're going to save and when as well as the final tally in your bank account at the end.

By quantifying your goal, you can define your progress. Even while writing this book, I can't help looking at how much I have written for the day. You might feel like the end is far away or that you haven't done enough, but by tracking your progress, you immediately have facts that help you stay motivated. This is very important in keeping your spirit up when you feel you can't see the beginning of your journey of achievement—or the end.

This lack of vision and progress can be very discouraging when climbing a mountain. When I first climbed to the Mount Everest base camp, the beginning was horrible. Looking up at the mountain was discouraging enough but hearing how long it was going to take was even worse (let alone the story about dead bodies in the mountain!).

But once you take the first few steps and start looking back, something invigorates you. You feel this rush of energy as you see how far you have travelled. *I've come too far to stop now.*

You keep going.

Seeing your progress keeps you striving for your goal.

Another benefit is that as you look at how long you have left till you achieve your goal, you realize that things are becoming possible. What may have seemed like an impossible task is becoming achievable. That feeling is uplifting and will actually encourage you to finish it.

When you can see the finish line, you keep going
because you know it's almost over.

For me, that experience was seeing the end of my team's virtual reality project, Crazy Fishing VR. The game had come a long way, but it didn't feel like we were progressing. We were close to giving up. When we decided to actually play the game it was only then that we realized just how far we had come. We noticed the things we had made, like the detailed fishes and the mini-games.

Seeing what you have made and what you have left to do helps enormously. So, keep track of your progress!

Once you know your progress, you will know how fast or slow you've been working relative to your deadline. Knowing this will allow you to adjust accordingly if you're falling behind your goal's time frame. This is another reason you must set a hard deadline.

When my friend, Thi, was competing for a triathlon, he noticed he was going too slow in his training. He practiced running and cycling, but not the third component: swimming. He didn't have much time left to practice, so he considered his training options and doubled down on swimming along the beaches of Australia (he's crazy!). I'm proud to say he completed that triathlon like a boss.

Don't set lame-ass arbitrary numbers though. For example, if you want to lose (or gain) weight, don't just pull a number out of thin air. Consider your current weight and a realistic number of pounds. Then set your progress according to that number.

To go into further detail, make the progress *real*. Let's go back to the digging tunnel analogy. You could *fake* progress by saying that every day you will pick up the shovel 50 times! That sounds great, but you're getting nowhere. Instead, you need to say that you will pick up the shovel full of dirt 50 times to make that tunnel. This might sound silly, but many frustrated achievers do this, myself included.

A common example I find with fake progress is when people learn a language. There is nothing wrong with learning new words, but at some point, you need to tackle grammar and how to form a sentence. Instead, they continue learning new words, without making any real progress toward actually speaking the language.

Or perhaps you want to expand your cake business. Instead of just calling 10 random people per day to ask them if they will buy your cakes, why not target 10 industry-related or carefully researched people?

You must track real progress.

A huge component people miss is reviewing what they have done.

You must get in the habit of looking at your progress on a schedule, every time, at the same time, in relation to your deadlines. There will be days that the tracking seems discouraging, like the days when I look to see that I have done nothing.

Jerry Seinfeld, an extremely successful comedian, circled every day on a calendar when he created a new joke. Soon, he no longer wanted to break the chain of circles.

This kind of momentum will help push you through your goals.

So, you can't achieve your goals if you don't track how the hell they are doing. With a scorecard that can act as your reference point, you can keep yourself motivated and directed. When times get hard, look back at what you've done so far and how much is left to go.

And when things get easy, know that you can do a lot more. Achievement is only attainable when you measure your progress. You can't blindly dig a tunnel. You don't just run faster. You can't lose weight without measuring what you eat.

If you want to actually achieve shit, quantify your progress.

20. YOU HATE THE BORING SHIT

Do you really think athletes find it enjoyable to run the same distances over and over again, just to shave a few seconds off their time? Or actors love working out in the gym day in and day out to get the physique they need for their role? The harsh truth is: *no.*

No one loves the mundane stuff. Heck, the definition of boring is exactly that: boring.

['bôriNG]

adjective

1. not interesting; tedious.

"I've got a boring job in an office."

But what sets apart achievers from non-achievers is that they do the seriously boring shit that no one else does. And they do them because they know that these seemingly insignificant and boring actions add up.

If everyone were willing to do all the boring stuff, we would have a lot of achievers out there. But we don't. No one loves doing the same thing over and over again.

When I see programmers, I imagine sitting at a computer changing one number hoping to tune something to perfection. I'm bored even thinking about it.

There are countless things we consider boring but know are crucial to achieving what we want. The writer has to edit her book over and over until she is happy with it. The language learner needs to learn the alphabet. The podcast producer needs to fine tune and listen to their podcast until it's perfect. The takeaway: All the boring stuff is necessary.

I was fortunate to talk to a Twitch/YouTube streamer who was very successful. He told me that everyone thinks he's having fun playing computer games, but behind the scenes, he has to edit his videos and create new types of content.

Even when making my own content, editing videos is more of a chore, at least to me. The reality is that no matter what you want to achieve, there will be boring parts—you cannot avoid them. You must admit and accept that they are part of the plan. If you get them done now, the further you move toward achieving your goals.

But what happens if we leave the boring things out? I tried that too many times for me to count.

When I had a concept to create an app that would show the free parking spots around Australia, I knew I was on to something. No app existed and I felt it was going to be the best idea ever. However, I needed to do two things: learn to program and walk around the city to label all the free parking spots. Learning to program is fun. It's a whole new language and it's very exciting—so, that's where I started—but also the place I stayed.

The problem was I loved programming so much I got sidetracked. I learned new things that weren't even necessary. When I tried to do the other half of my project—walk around the city to find the free parking spots—I got bored and would rush home to program.

What happened in the end? Well, even if I was the best programmer in the world, without the locations of all the free parking spots, what the fuck did I really have?

Months went by and I just didn't want to go out and map out free parking spots. It's boring to walk around just to map things. Some days, I just stopped and played computer games. At times, I even forgot why I was learning to program. I just did what was fun. And I got nothing done.

I was fortunate though. I had one of those moments where I asked myself, "What are you doing with your life?" and decided to walk around the city like an absolute boss. I coded all the locations in and finished the app. I published it myself and was waiting for the money to come in. It did not.

A few months later, a company approached me to buy the data points. I had no idea why, but any money was welcomed, and I sold it all for $2000. Yes, around six months of work got me $2000. I probably earned thirty-cents per hour. But for me, this was an achievement. It taught me that the boring stuff is necessary to finish your goals—and it might just be the moneymaker. More importantly though, it made me realize I was capable of creating something from nothing. Wouldn't it be great to get paid to just sit and do what you enjoyed the most? But to achieve shit, this is not possible. I've seen people simply quit because things just got boring.

One friend ran for a few weeks, and then quit because he felt "running was boring" even though his goal was to complete a marathon.

Another friend wanted to become an investment banker but felt looking at financial data and making slide decks was boring. There are boring components to everything you want to do. It won't always be fun, so stop looking for it to be. Just do what you have to do.

I'm not here to sap your energy and say that fun things can't be productive. They certainly can be, and fun is also a vital component to what you want. But the barrier everyone faces, most of all, is the boring shit. It's why people try to make the boring stuff fun.

Multiple apps already exist that make boring things into games. For example, there's exercising for points where good habits are created by tracking your "score." You can learn coding by making games and battling other people. There are many ways to make things more enjoyable, but you can't make everything fun.

Think of achievement as a mix of both fun and boring. You can concentrate on the fun and get half of the stuff done, but then all you are left with is the boring crap. So, try to find the stuff that bores you and add some of the fun stuff in.

For example, when I exercise, I add in music or different types of exercise to make it more enjoyable. I cook different foods to add variety even though I am on a strict diet. When I program, I do the boring code, then spend a few minutes playing with my actual app.

You need to be creative. If you can't find any fun at all – well then, looks like you consumed all the fun and it's time you sit down and face the boring shit.

Deal with the boring stuff and you will achieve what you want.

21. YOU READY, AIM, AND NEVER FIRE

This is how you do *not* achieve your goals.

You research what is necessary to obtain your goals. You prepare what is necessary and mentally get ready for the journey ahead. You start to visualize your goals. You know where you plan to go and how you will get there. If there's going to be a mistake or an error where you might screw up, you change the plan. You revise and perfect it. Rinse and repeat.

Then you get old.

You die.

You didn't execute because there was a chance of error.

You aim so much you don't ever fire.

Just take the fucking shot. It doesn't matter if you miss.

I was always aiming but never firing. Readying yourself is easy. Aiming is just as easy. And with the abundant amount of material available on the Internet, it's easy to continually aim and never take the shot.

What stops us is the fear to fail. To protect ourselves from that fear, we want everything to be perfect. I have felt that I needed to have the perfect plan. That way I would prevent any failures and, hence, I wouldn't be disappointed in myself.

But as anyone who has actually obtained their goals will tell you, there *will* be failure and mistakes. The difference is you're often allowed to fire again. You don't need to be perfect.

Does it really matter how long you take aim?

When you hold off for too long, you could miss the wave. This happened to me when I first started developing for smartphones.

The iPhone had just come out (yes, the very first one) and it was a game changer. Apps were new and they were hot. Anyone who made a remotely decent app had a good chance of succeeding. I felt I had an idea that was going to be awesome, so I spent a year trying to figure out how my app was going to work. I planned for a long time, and by the time I was ready to even start learning to develop, it was the third generation of iPhones.

The field had been reset, everything was changing, and I was left behind. I would have been in a better position to succeed if I had just started. Getting an app out earlier was a huge advantage and I gave that chance up.

So, how do you start to achieve your goals?

You do a little research, mentally prepare for what you needed to do, admit it's going to take a long time—and know you can't give up. You set a clear target on what you are aiming for. You get ready to take the next step. Then, just go fucking in!

Go as far as you can till you make a mistake. Re-aim and fire again. The faster you fire the better. You can make mistakes. It's part of the process. Naysayers will say, *I don't want to go in blindly!* You won't. You still aim. You still prepare. You just don't make perfection your goal. You must fire at some point or die aiming.

A person aiming for a target must take time to determine why they missed. Revise mistakes and errors. Then get ready to fire again.

You might convince yourself that you only have one shot at something. But really, you get as many shots as you want until you give up.

My friend Alex was adamant on getting an MBA. He put everything into his first attempt and got rejected from all the schools he applied to. He convinced himself that it was over, and his goals were no longer achievable. So, he gave up.

He spent the next year saying he had no direction in life and no idea where to go. But something gnawed at him and he ended up applying again to his one dream school—and got rejected once again.

Long story short, he did eventually get into his dream school—the year after. He wasted a year thinking of his application and acting as if the world was over. He ended up wasting two years. He stopped firing. He thought that after one shot it was done.

One day he even asked me to open a letter for him to see if he got rejected. I don't believe in prayers, but if there was any time I was praying, it was there and then.

Time is short. You can't stand around thinking you lost it all on one shot. You can't spend years aiming. You will die with regret. The fewer shots you take, the fewer chances you have at actually succeeding. So, don't spend all your life aiming and preparing.

Time is short.

You can't waste it on thinking you lost it all with one shot.

You can't spend years aiming and not firing.

Take your shots.

Don't die regretting that you didn't.

22. YOU NEVER FINISH
WHAT YOU START

Has a friend ever told you that he's going to do something and never ends up doing it? He has these goals and never ends up meeting them. You may be the same. The scariest part of all is that it can become a habit.

You create a habit of never finishing what you start.

I used to be just like that. Overpromise and never deliver.

When I look back at those times, I realize I was pretending I could achieve things. I was trying to make myself look good but, in the end, I shot myself in the foot. At first, people will believe you. They want to believe you can do it.

But the more you say what you plan to do, the harder it gets for you. You risk meeting people who don't want you to succeed or people who divert you away from your goals. You add pressure to yourself unnecessarily. If you collapse under that pressure you will fail to achieve your goals and people will remember that.

People may ask how your project is going. You might respond with a nothing or just shrug it off. Fewer people will believe you can do it, and you end up crushing yourself.

During my university days, a friend, Mike, always told me about his grandiose plan to build an app that would change the world. It was actually a messaging app that was fully private with messages that would delete after a specified time. Every time he was at parties, he would say how useful it was going to be, giving examples such as sending important messages or showing off places with a time limit.

One day, in front of a few friends he said, "It's going to happen." But it never did—and we got tired of hearing that it would.

Friends would say, "Mike, it's not happening, just forget the idea." He would get defensive and argue that he was going to do it.

Then, months later, Snapchat came out. It did exactly what Mike described his app would do. Mike never made anything and went silent after that.

I was the same. I told people how I planned to create an empire. My vision was to build a specialist medical clinic comprising of different people and skills that would complement each other.

What happened? Nothing. I got nowhere. When a colleague decided to point out to me that I never achieved my goal, I felt angry. But I deserved it. I never did what the fuck I said I would do. Every time I failed to complete something it reminded me that maybe I could never get my goals done at all.

I just started giving up. *I can't achieve anything. I might as well just do nothing at all.* This was shitty thinking.

That's not to say you can't tell people what your vision may be. But if you can't handle the pressure, be the person who does it in silence. It is far more respectable if you only let people see your results. If you do choose to tell people what your plans are, make sure those you tell can keep you accountable for your goals. They will encourage you to finish or at least support you along your journey.

If you don't finish what you start, then trust and opportunities will fade away. Who would you hire, a person who has successfully developed and shipped multiple apps or a person who can't even finish one?

The things you accomplish *do* matter. Even if it's your personal goals, achieving them will be a reflection of who you are: a person who gets shit done.

It is amazing what opportunities come to people who actually finish their goals.

Jason, a developer working at one of my companies, had made multiple games in his free time. None of these games made any money, mind you. I hired him because of his portfolio alone, but he had no degree. He taught himself programming and just made some fun stuff. Eventually, we had to let Jason go. Why? Because he got an offer at Google, as a developer. He got picked up by a recruiter who saw his achievements.

Before he left, we had a chat. He told me that even when he felt like just stopping, he reminded himself that he was programming for a reason: to create fun games for himself and his friends. And if he never finished a game, it would never be played. That idea kept him motivated to finish what he started.

You must always go back to the root of why you created your goal in the first place and why you would ever consider not finishing it. By finishing your goals, people will believe in your ideas and see you as a person who can make things actually happen. With that reputation, opportunities may come to you that allow you to continue to achieve newer and greater things.

The point is this: Finish the shit you start. Otherwise, don't bother starting.

23. YOU DON'T SWEAT
THE SMALL STUFF

We often think that small things don't matter.

How can reading one page in a book amount to anything? How can jogging for five minutes do anything for my health? If the small stuff doesn't matter, then why bother doing them?

Big goals require millions of little things that just seem so insignificant. Reading one page in a gigantic book, pfft! Why bother?

Yet how on earth do you plan to save hundreds of dollars, if you can't save one dollar? How do you plan to be super fit if you don't lift a single weight?

It all starts with one.

I had never made a video until I actually started recording.

Purchasing a video camera didn't get me started. Downloading a video editor didn't help. I needed to start somewhere and that was by pressing the record button on my video camera.

Even thinking of making a video scared the crap out of me. I didn't think it would be possible. When I actually got in front of the camera it took me ages to be happy with something I had recorded.

Then, I looked at loading it on the editor and just decided to stop.

I could predict how long it would take—a damn long time—so I left the footage there, unedited. When I finally pushed myself to get it done, it was by far the worst video I had ever seen.

But even so, it helped me understand the process. I learned how to make better footage and how to do editing far quicker and more effectively. This taught me to be much more efficient later in video production. All these little actions helped me produce videos in the future.

It's the small things that matter. When I wanted to clean my house, I started with a small corner. It didn't feel like much at first, but over the course of time that clean corner turned into a clean room and eventually into a clean house. It's much like a little snowball. It's tiny at first, but as it rolls down the hill it accumulates more snow. It gets bigger and bigger until it becomes something that can make a difference.

When I first went to the gym, I had no idea how all the equipment worked. I had poor technique and was honestly shy about picking up weights and using them in front of other people. But as I spent more time going to the gym, I was able to learn from other gym goers on how to use the equipment. I started to become more confident and comfortable. None of that was possible unless I took the first step.

It really just takes one step.

It is very easy to rationalize that one step means nothing. It gives you no visual change or indication of how much you have improved. It's why I recommend listening to Admiral McRaven's "Make Your Bed" speech, which was later turned into a book.

A simple thing, such as making your bed, may not seem like much, but it starts your day off realizing you can do one thing and finish it. When I started going on an exercise rampage, I felt I was making no progress even though I was exercising and dieting like crazy. For weeks, I had been going hard and had nothing to show for it.

But after six weeks something happened. I looked at photos and noticed my own reflection. *Holy crap!* I don't have a one-pack but a two-pack! Something was forming. When I was about to give up, something started to show. It didn't have to be huge, but it was *something*.

I have always wondered how an old friend of mine, Ellen, rocked the absolute dance floor at a wedding. I wondered how a girl who was clumsy and had fallen over at one of our school assemblies managed to dance like a pro.

When I was fortunate enough to talk to her, she told me she practiced every day. She was in tears after that assembly and I don't blame her (I remember laughing at her, too). It motivated her to practice again and again. Some days she was in tears because nothing would work. But things changed when she went to a dance class to assess her level. Her teacher immediately told her to jump to intermediate classes.

She was shocked. *"But I'm not that good,"* she told the teacher. Her teacher made her perform in front of a class. Nervous and sweating, she did a dance to Hyuna's Bubble Pop (a K-pop song). A round of applause followed her dance that led Ellen to continually dance her heart out.

You must always start somewhere. It doesn't matter where or how tiny it may be—you do it. Study just one extra word in French.

Run one extra mile.

Do one extra rep lifting weights.

No matter how small that may be to you, it's still something.

How do you plan to achieve something if you don't even take a single step forward? Similar to the tortoise and the hare, it is far better to take a step in the direction you want to go than to dance around playing games because you're so sure you will get it done.

Every step counts.
Every little action you do contributes to your goal.
Don't ever think what you do is pointless or not worth it.
It is.
Everything fucking counts.

24. YOU WANT A MAGIC BULLET

Thinking of taking a shortcut? Finding the fastest way possible? In a very entrepreneurial society, it would seem everyone knows better than everyone else.

How is this possible?

For some reason, we sometimes think we are *better* than people who have achieved things. The people who have achieved their goals took a very long path, and a very painful one, too. They tell us exactly how to get there, but we just don't listen. They tell us it takes time and discipline. What do we do? We throw it right out the window and try to find the fastest way to get there with absolute disregard to the people that made it in the first place.

We search for shortcuts. We try to find magic bullets.

I know magic bullets may seem to work. You know, the guy on the infomercial with a giant eight-pack telling you that this magical machine is going to give you abs "like these"!

Or take a look at that well-dressed person showing you how to make heaps of money for only $99! We want to believe that there is a shortcut that will lead us to success. But if every fucking shortcut worked, how come we don't see an abundance of achievers? Where the hell are they? They don't exist because shortcuts don't work.

That's not to say I haven't dabbled in shortcuts. I wished they worked, too. When I was naive, one program I fell victim to was those make-money-fast packages.

These online cons start off strong, convincing you that their program will show you how to make a fuck-load of money. I felt good about my purchase, but then found that the material was rehashing the same stuff over and over again. It then told me to get another package and a whole bunch of other crap.

I realized by the end of the first part of the program that I knew nothing, and it had taught me only the absolute basics.

But let me reveal the magic it taught me: Buy an item from China. Put a brand on it. Buy ads on Amazon. Sell it on Amazon. Ta-da! Magic. The magic is called drop-shipping. Don't fall for this shit.

You don't achieve anything by shortcuts.

Shortcuts are a great selling point though. They make you feel like you're doing something even when you aren't. The amount of time you put into them goes nowhere. You will invest your resources into a shortcut only to end up learning that it doesn't work. Eight weeks to learn programming. Six months to get a degree. The thought of time saved has definitely won me over a few times.

Then, I realized all the shortcuts were simply distractions from the long road ahead.

When I had finished a small programming course that "equipped" me with the fundamentals, I got nowhere. I felt I could program, but when it got down to doing real work, I couldn't do a single thing. I had no idea how to tackle an actual task.

It's like learning the alphabet and then being told to write a novel.

My 'Aha' moment in programming was when I directed it into a project I wanted to get done. And no shortcut was going to help.

I had to find the answers to the specific questions tailored to the project. The learning process of solving my own specific problems taught me far more than any other magic bullet could.

It's the gritty learning processes that will equip you to achieve the shit you want. You can't skip the hard work. Sooner or later it will come and bite you.

We live in an age where "hacks" are an obsession—little tricks to make things easier. We use these little gimmicks to reduce time and effort to achieve our goals, but there are no shortcuts to success. If there were, we would all be successful. However, last time I checked, only a handful of people seem to be achieving shit.

There's no damn substitute for hard work.

You need to be realistic about how long your goals will take. Don't try to cheat the system. If some secret passageway existed, some person would have figured it out—and they probably wouldn't share it with you, either!

So, if someone tells you a shortcut exists, forget it. Don't waste time chasing shortcuts that get you nowhere.

I actually made fun of an ex-friend for learning how to play piano the hard way. All he did was play hard pieces over and over again. When he couldn't do something, he looked up how to play it via YouTube. He had no teacher or guidance. He just learned.

Now he can play piano by just looking at a piece and impress people at parties. I'm jealous.

So, fuck you, shortcuts.

25. YOU DON'T STICK TO ONE GOAL

How many goals do you have? If you had to choose only one goal, which one would it be?

You have so many goals and you want to achieve them all. So do I. So do your friends and family. We all want to do so much shit that we get nothing done.

You achieve nothing by doing multiple things at once. Do one thing well and concentrate on it 100%.

The issue with having multiple goals is the false sense of progression it can give you. The moment something gets difficult, you stop working on that project and move on to another project. You haven't technically given up, because you haven't truly stopped (this is called rationalizing). You are just making a detour.

Now you work on the new goal until that gets hard. Now where do you go? You go to one of your other goals on the list. The difficult parts pile up and you keep jumping around. The fear or the hard work that's required just doesn't feel great, so you finally give up.

Then you ask yourself why the fuck aren't you getting anything done.

Let me share with you something stupid I have done.

I tried studying Mandarin and Cantonese at the same time. When Mandarin got hard, I jumped into learning some basic words in Cantonese. When Cantonese got hard, I went back to Mandarin. I was bouncing back and forth. I did this for a whole fucking year.

I have no doubt my girlfriend at the time was frustrated hearing me jump from one goal to the next. I ended up wasting time because I could barely speak either language in the end. After dropping Mandarin completely and going in guns blazing with Cantonese, I achieved conversational fluency in a year (I picked Cantonese in the end; for those who are wondering, it's just a lot more fun).

When I look back on my idiocy of jumping between two languages, I realize it was because when Mandarin got hard, I could jump to something easier.

Learning the alphabet, doing light weights at the gym, or planning out a business idea is the easy part. It also gives you a sense of progress. But really, you're just avoiding the hard things.

The difficult parts are the most important steps in obtaining your goals. They are also the ones that feel crappy doing.

But you must do them.

By having only one goal, you have to face these difficult hurdles—you have nowhere else to jump to—and that restriction may seem horrible at first, but it's the only way you can achieve at least one goal on your list.

When you concentrate on multiple goals, it's inevitable that you will fail to achieve them. How can you say did everything you could?

Failure will only be justified if you do *your very best*.

Imagine failing to be an actor because you forgot your lines, all because you were so busy cramming for your medical exams. If you are going to pursue something, just fucking pursue one "something." If one fails because you were trying to do something else, the regret will eat at you forever.

I have had a friend fail a consulting interview because she was up the night before learning how to program. Concentrating on too many things is dangerous because it can cost you great opportunities and can also lead you down the road to failure.

Mind you, concentrating on one goal is extremely difficult. I couldn't do it for years. And year after year you start to promise yourself that *this* year will be different. But it never changes, and nothing happens. You don't move forward.

At the beginning of the year, you have ambitious goals, multiple goals, and in the end, you get none of them done. If you can't get *one* done, how can you get all the other shit on your list done? At least when you reflect on your efforts, you can say you got *one* finished.

At least complete one thing. Forget multiple goals, just do one and finish it.

When you actually complete one goal, it will give you momentum. It helps you realize that you're capable of achieving what you set out to do. That's a mindset that helps you achieve larger goals. The more difficult the goal, the greater the momentum.

When I finished a marathon (in a very poor time, 5:34 by the way), I felt completing *anything* was possible.

What else can I do? What other goals have I missed out on?

That momentum is impossible to create unless you have achieved your goal. So, complete one of your goals at a time.

When I briefly lived in Hong Kong, I met Phan, a computer science graduate. Like many graduates, he had no idea what to do. He tried data science and mobile game development. His reasoning was that one paid the bills and the other was a hobby.

I thought it was fairly reasonable until he started to juggle them religiously: a bit of data science here, a bit of game programming there. The problem was that when he had an interview for one of the two, he wouldn't get the job because he didn't have the depth of knowledge required.

Unexpectedly, he threw out data science and went deep into game development. He produced a few mobile games and got a job in an indie game development studio. This year I heard news that he was moving to Korea to help run a new game company, as a partner.

If you want to achieve, you must concentrate on one thing.

There is no equal priority for your goals. I could never say I wanted two things equally. You will want one more than the other, If you don't, flip a coin— and that's going to be it. No more switching.

Stick to one goal and finish it.

PART III

YOUR SURROUNDINGS

What you surround yourself with matters.
Your environment can affect you.

26. YOU SPEND TIME COMPARING

It is human nature to compare. Without a comparison how do we know where we are at in our life? Are we behind or in front? Is this book better than the one I read before?

I love comparing.

If I compare to people who have achieved far more than me, it can motivate me. Yet other times, these comparisons will crush me, giving me extreme ideas about how far I am or should be in my life. Most of the time, it's just better to avoid comparisons because none are realistic.

The most dangerous comparisons involve using factors that just can't be changed. *That person is richer than me. She is more attractive. He is so lucky.* These comparisons don't help and usually make us feel worse off.

When you compare yourself or your efforts to something that can't be changed, you run into a wall because of that lack of control.

Remember, you can only change yourself.

If you fall into the trap of comparing things that cannot be changed, you begin to feed into your excuses as to why these people are better than you. You can fall into an endless cycle of despair. So, you need to accept that the world is just like that. Some people are born beautiful. Some people are born rich. You can't change that.

But you *can* work on yourself.

I had a friend who would compare himself to other people incessantly. When a mutual friend of ours had profited off the cryptocurrency bubble, he would say that our friend was just lucky.

But what he didn't know was that when bitcoin was $50, our friend was eating only cans of tuna to buy more bitcoin. He believed in it.

At the time of this writing, the rate of exchange is $10,000 for each bitcoin. I'm glad he succeeded in making some money.

Did my friend feel that way? Nope. He just kept saying our friend was lucky. He just kept wishing he could have what our friend had. He no longer looked at what he could do in his *own* situation. Instead, he only looked at what *others* had.

We can't change the fortunes or misfortunes of others; all we can really do is change ours.

You can't achieve anything unless you stop comparing.

Everyone is different. You can't compare yourself to someone similar in age, as maturity levels are different. You can't even compare to people with the same college degree and background, because their parents are different. These are fruitless endeavors that will lead you nowhere. Everyone is unique. Different life situations create different paths.

I have a couple friends who are doctors, Markus and David. David sped through studying medicine as rapidly as possible. Markus did the same. But Markus fell in love—and this is where their paths split.

Markus ended up marrying a woman whose family in China was well off. The family welcomed him and gave him a new life. Markus is now happily running multiple clinics, and last time I saw him, he was driving a new Ferrari.

But what happened to David? David graduated and also fell in love. But his life turned out the absolute reverse of Markus's. He's divorced; has been upset for years; becoming bitter and seems to just go through life like it is one giant struggle.

Markus made me think that becoming a doctor would make me rich. David made me feel like becoming a doctor was a bad idea. But both are stupid thoughts, right? Their eventual circumstances had nothing to do with being a doctor.

But this is what we do when we compare ourselves to other people.

What happens in someone's life is an unknown. The person we compare ourselves to at a very specific moment in time is a poor reflection of what they have been or will go through. You are comparing yourself to a highlight reel or an Instagram photo.

I remember looking at a photo of a friend in Bali. You know those people who just seem to have an endless supply of money? That was him. He had photos with celebrities, women hanging from him and an infinite amount of drinks. The comparisons in my mind began.

At first, I started to compare myself. *Man, he's got it all. Why don't I have that? Wait, is that Brad Pitt? I need a dog in my photos. I can never get that rich. He doesn't deserve this. I should have...* And I started to hate myself.

But I had forgotten one thing: At one time, this guy was poor.

I remember a day when he had to sleep on my couch because he had no place to stay. He was broke and homeless, and his parents wanted nothing to do with him. We only hung around for a few days, but he always told me about organic food. He knew everything there was about it. At the time, I didn't care. Food was food.

But he had an idea and, a few years later, he executed his business idea and became the supplier for farm fresh food.

Remembering all this, I swiped down on my Instagram to see the next photo and thought to myself, *Man, he deserves it.*

Comparisons to anyone today is simply denying all the work they did to get to where they are. Imagine comparing the present-day Richard Branson to yourself now. He's rich, philanthropic, and very successful. But what about all the hardships he went through? The times he was in jail? The failures he went through with his company?

We make assumptions that don't help ourselves or anyone else. We just don't know. And those assumptions just make us feel like we can't ever achieve what we want.

The people you make assumptions about got there because they deserved it. You can make it and deserve it, too.

Since you are the one consistent variable in any equation,
you can continually work to improve yourself.

If you didn't run today, run now. If you failed to work on your goals yesterday, work on your goals today. If you didn't achieve anything yesterday, achieve something today.

This is the only comparison that you will need to make:
yesterday's version of yourself to today's version.

27. YOU AREN'T SELFISH ENOUGH

"Being selfish is bad."

When I was younger, I would agree. Being selfish meant you didn't give a fuck about other people. But there is a very thin line between being selfish and not being selfish.

If you help someone else out, doesn't it make them selfish and you selfless? If your friend told you to help them with their goal, wouldn't *that* be selfish? If you ever want to achieve your goals and dreams, you *have* to be selfish, especially with your time.

I have a friend who is a consistent giver. She continually gives up her own time for others. It makes her feel good and she feels like she's contributing to society. But, personally, she hasn't achieved much.

She does have a lot of personal goals such as running a café, but she continuously puts these activities aside for other people. *Their* goals take priority over *her* own goals.

I have no doubt she feels great helping people, but often she would grudgingly tell people she couldn't pursue her own goals because she has no time. Her world has become full of people willing to take advantage of her generosity.

Your priorities, goals, and dreams should come first. I'm certainly not suggesting you stomp on everyone who is in your way. But you must respect *your* own time. Sure, help others, but your priority should always be your own goals. They are yours and you are responsible for them.

There are people willing to blame others for their failure to succeed. When they can't achieve their dreams, they will point the finger to someone else. *I had to help my brother. I had to help my friends move. I had to help arrange my friend's birthday party.*

If you have excuses, you can justify failing to achieve what you want.

When I was younger, a girl I had been dating was always telling me to go out on dates with her. I got angry and blamed her for not giving me the time to work on my own shit.

But the moment I said it, regret rushed through me.

I blamed her when I should have blamed myself. I *chose* to go on those dates. I *chose* to spend time with her. It was not her responsibility but my own.

If you have no stake in your goals, how will you learn from the failures?

You can hand it off to someone else.

Imagine playing golf and hitting the ball so far that it misses the hole completely. You could blame the wind. You could blame the sun glaring in your eyes. But you learn nothing from all that blaming.

It's the same with helping others. *You* decided to help your friend. Countless times I have seen people throw up their hands and blame their parents or friends, and then justify how they "tried" to pursue their goals.

You can't learn if you don't become selfish in your pursuit of achievement. By being selfish, you blame only yourself.

A few years ago, I tried to be extremely helpful to people. I wasn't sure what to do, so I decided to help those around me. I queued up my schedule with everything: helping my friends develop a website, supporting my friends study group, and doing pro-bono consulting work. By the end of the year, I felt good about helping people, but none of *my* goals were achieved.

When I withdrew my help from others, I received insults and was told I was not "nice."

It is easy to convince yourself that no hard feelings will happen just by you being nice and helping friends. Yet, when you make a change and withdraw your help, people won't be happy about it. Perhaps you have told your friends that you can't help them because you have something else to do, something in pursuit of your goals. Maybe you can't assist your family because you have an interview for your dream job. Whatever the case, when you actually put your foot down and aren't as available, they will label you as selfish.

Don't let the guilt they try to dish out overcome you. If they really cared about your goals, they would understand.

When I first decided to become selfish, I felt like shit. I bailed on a friend's birthday party because I had a choice between the party and working with one of my app developers. I made the choice to work on releasing the app. Do I regret it? Not at all.

Life is full of choices and you need to make the choice that suits you, not others.

But it's at times like these that you will know who your friends really are. A few told me I was the worst friend in the world. Maybe. A few others told me they would have done the same. Those who really care about you will want to see you succeed. You don't lose out on anything if you actually hold your ground to reach that success.

You are responsible for your own life.

So, before you go to help someone or think you need to be somewhere to avoid hard feelings, remember your dreams and goals.

You want to live a life that is fulfilling to you—and achieving what you want does that. There's nothing wrong with being selfish, if you plan to achieve what you want.

You can't compromise on your dreams.

You can't be pushed over by other people who care for themselves and likely have far different goals than you.

Your goals are yours. To achieve them you must be selfish.

28. YOU HAVE TOXIC FRIENDS

Is your friendship or relationship doing you more harm than good?

Toxic relationships are the worst.

Why would you have someone stick around who is doing you harm? This harm could be mental, such as the girl who makes fun of you in public or the guy who seems to be putting you down every time you have a great idea.

Why do we keep people around us who are clearly horrible for us?

The answer: what we have invested in the relationship.

Sometimes the relationship formed when we were young. We keep these friendships because we have invested many years of energy into the relationship. You hold onto it even though that person has changed.

People change. They mature.

They change their direction in life, or they just no longer like the same things you do. Yet even when our directions and lives differ greatly, we *still* hold onto these friendships. The other person may no longer support you or care for you anymore—and contact with them brings you down. But, you endure your toxic relationships because your time investment has made them a part of your life—and you cannot figure out how to end it.

An unfortunate example would be my ex-best friend, Joel.

We had studied together throughout high school and university, and then, Joel started to change.

He started to dislike "winners." I have no idea where this mindset came from, but every time someone succeeded, he made passing remarks such as "he doesn't deserve it" or "what a showoff." These jabs took a toll on a few friends and me.

My personal exposure to his toxic-ness was when I got my first successful funding for a start-up. The first thing Joel said was, "You shouldn't do it. You will waste their money."

I turned to him, and said, "Fuck off, man."

It felt horrible at first but, all of a sudden, I felt freer. It was a great relief and the shackles were off.

This is not to say people with different directions shouldn't be your friends. On the contrary, some of our best friends are the very opposite of us. But when the directions become harmful to us, we must consider if they will deter us from our goals.

If people around you become toxic in your life, they are not worth it. If you can burn the bridge, burn it. Get rid of them immediately. They are worthless obstacles. Do not let one person's toxic outlook on life stop you from getting what you want.

I know sometimes it isn't possible to do a clean cut-off. Perhaps the relationship exists out of pure necessity. You can't just leave your parents, your siblings, your boss or even your colleagues. You can't leave them straight away. It's unrealistic.

Sometimes a person who has been spurned will come back with a vengeance. Look at the actions of Sam Walton, who founded Walmart. A business associate had kicked him out of his original shop location and took over the business he had grown. Years later, Walton built a Walmart near that shop and put the man out of business. His intent wasn't to ruin the man, the location was still a prime spot after all, but the result is all the same.

You don't know what will happen in relationships that have become toxic to you.

If you're concerned about burning a bridge, stop maintaining it.

When you stop maintaining the toxic relationship, does the relationship go south? Or does it simply fade away?

When you stop tending to a toxic relationship, you really find out who actually cares. The relationships that were meant to fade will simply do just that. It's a two-way street. It shouldn't be one person holding it all together, but both of you.

You will sometimes feel that it's wrong, but life is too short to waste further time on relationships that won't work. People who aren't supportive and detract you from achieving your dreams and your goals are a waste of time and energy.

It's frightening how often people are willing to hold onto toxic relationships, even though they know it's bad for them. I have seen friends let a person treat them like absolute shit and discourage them from doing anything productive.

A good friend of mine, Stacey, does favors for friends just because they ask. But when she needed help, no one was there for her. They used her, but she kept holding on. The scariest thing is that Stacey could never see how they didn't support her or her goals.

When she wanted to work on her own little cupcake stall, the friends she had helped told her it was a silly idea. When she was learning new ways to decorate cakes, these same friends asked her to help with groceries. Yes, fucking groceries.

She could have said no, but her friends knew what she was doing and set up obstacles, prioritizing something they wanted.

Stacey always said yes.

Stacey won't achieve anything so long as these people are around.

Toxic people will prevent you from achieving anything.

The age-old saying is that you are the average of the people you hang around most. If you hang around toxic people, you will attract toxic people, because you are likely to become toxic.

It also happens the other way around.

As you remove these bad relationships from your world, the better you become. And more importantly, higher quality people will find you. These people will push you in the right direction and help you achieve what you want. When you have achievers around you, you will feel the drive to achieve more. You will be pulled *up* not down.

One of the greatest changes I saw concerning toxicity was in one of my developers who used to work for me. Lionel had a friend called Adrian.

Adrian was a liar, and absolutely toxic. He pulled Lionel out to party and do drugs. Every time Lionel wanted to do work, Adrian would tell him it was a waste of time. Consequently, Lionel came to work late every day and was not productive.

Later, Lionel quit to work on a project with Adrian (Adrian convinced him it was not good to work with my team).

That's where shit got messy.

Adrian would make Lionel do all the work and justified this by saying that he was always taking Lionel out to parties. Once the project was complete, Adrian ran away with it and all the money.

Lionel was left with nothing and he had to fend for himself. His best friend had betrayed him, and he felt used. But he learned a powerful lesson about toxicity. Although the next year was tough, he started to find time for himself.

Time alone is far better than hanging with a toxic friend.

Lionel found a small job to keep him afloat and meet new people. Although I have not seen him since, I have checked his recent activities and was happy to see a photo of him and his new girlfriend. He's out there with his own goals and I hope he achieves them.

Your energy and devotion should be directed to the most important people in your life. The people who make you better and challenge you in a positive way. They should be supportive, not consuming every trickle of time you have for yourself.

No one deserves toxicity. You must concentrate on building good relationships and not tolerating or maintaining bad ones.

Toxic people will prevent you from achieving what you want.

Don't let toxicity be the reason you can't achieve shit you want.

29. YOU WASTE TIME THINKING OF REVENGE

When I sold my first medical clinic, the buyer was super friendly. We had drinks together and I was happy to sell the clinic to him. We went through the sale process together and discussed how he was going to let me manage the clinic. From there, things went smooth. Too smooth.

You know the name of this chapter, so you know what's going to happen.

He had put in my contract that he could terminate my contract anytime with a four-week notice. When I planned a one-month holiday, he planned to terminate my contract the day I was to leave.

I remember it well.

He said he wanted to have a word with me, and we talked. All of a sudden, he said he was ending the contract. The worst part was that I could not work in the industry for two years after the contract was terminated. I was screwed.

Moral of the story? Read contracts really well—and more than once.

The problem was compounded by a resentment that I held on to.

I wanted to get revenge. I pursued lawyers and talked to colleagues and asked other business sellers their advice.

What did they say?

There's nothing I could do.

But it always gnawed at me. I felt betrayed and backstabbed.

And what was he doing? Expanding the business. Making more money.

Me? Jobless and drowning in my own anger.

Revenge would have been so sweet. But the more I concentrated on revenge, the more I was making it about him. And the less I was thinking about myself.

You won't achieve shit if you let revenge be the motivator in your life.

As a bystander, I was fortunate to witness revenge at its greatest. Stan had been fired from his job because a work mate said he was stealing from the till. But it so happened that the accuser, Kyle, was stealing and needed someone to be the scapegoat.

The company ended up firing Stan because cash was missing, and the accuser was a good friend with the boss. Stan was livid. To be fired was one thing, to be told he was stealing when he wasn't—that was just too much. He thought of egging Kyle's house or even slashing his car tires.

In the end he did nothing, and I am thankful he didn't.

Stan would forget all about it until four years later. He met Kyle once again, but on a different footing. Stan saw him looking for a job at his office.

What did Stan do?

He told the recruiters that Kyle was bad news. Kyle stole from shops and should never be recruited. He got his revenge.

That night, Stan took us out for drinks to tell us the news. He told us his story. Craziest thing of all, Kyle had no clue why he lost his job.

Years later, Stan told us something I'm sure plagued him for a long time. Kyle had committed suicide. Stan would never know if it was because of what he did, but he certainly felt responsible and has never really been the same since.

His ambition and drive fell because he was riddled with guilt. The game of revenge is a very dangerous one.

There will be people willing to backstab you and take you down. They will just see you as someone in the way. Whatever the reason, they wrong you and you want revenge. You won't achieve shit if you pursue it though.

Revenge means you give power to whoever wronged you, which means they are dictating your life, controlling how you feel and what you do. And with such feelings clogging your mind, you have no way to really achieve the shit you want.

I've been there.

For months, I stood around saying, *Oh well, I can't work for a couple years, I'm fucked.* I never thought of a solution and I never even tried. All I could think of was how I could get revenge.

I remember driving past the clinic and saying to myself, maybe I should just go in there and yell at him. Did I? Nope. I was already wasting time just driving by there.

Instead, I started to focus on myself. I found a job outside the city and a new business partner to create a company.

So, what happened to the guy who backstabbed me? Last year, the business had gone downhill. The premises are vacant, and I have no idea if or where the business moved. Several clients contacted me through my personal channels and I forwarded them to someone who could look after them.

"Success is the best revenge."

Take this often quoted saying and work on yourself. Forget the other person. Just be all about achieving the shit you want in your life. Take a step back after getting pushed over. Breathe.

Think of what you want in your life and concentrate on that.

Put the past behind you. It's okay to feel upset—no one likes being used or thrown out.

Take baby steps toward realizing what you want for yourself and keep your focus on you and no one else. When you are successful you can honestly do whatever the fuck you want. *Get there first.*

Once you start obtaining your goals I have no doubt you will not give one fuck about people who have wronged you in the past.

Leave revenge behind. Do a one-eighty and set your mind on other things—like your goals.

30. YOU LET PEOPLE INFLUENCE YOU

You are the person in the arena. You're sweating it out and doing the work. But you're surprised by how many people want to criticize you and tell you how to do things. They want to convince you that there's a better path. They want to laugh at you when you fail.

But then, how the hell do they know? They aren't in the arena. They're sitting on their butts in the audience. They're bystanders, just watching while you're working.

They should have no bearing and influence on you.

I have been influenced by multiple people when I should have ignored them. "You aren't running your business properly! You should do this!" "You are doing a shitty job!" "You aren't trying hard enough!"

People love to throw their opinions around as though they're the ones in the arena.

You are the one sleeping less because your project is due tomorrow. *You* are the one sweating out at the gym trying to get fit. *You* are the one who is waking up early to create a business plan.

They don't know shit.

No one is immune to an audience yelling, but you mustn't listen to them. They may pretend to know everything, but they don't. Much like a sports fan who watches a game and thinks he can shoot a goal.

They have *no idea* how much work you have to put in. It's why when you're pursuing your goals, you must do so with conviction.

You can't allow the crowd to influence your direction.

You've probably witnessed this kind of mob mentality yourself. You might have seen parents tell their children to stop wasting their time pursuing useless things. Or heard a best friend who thinks their friend's hard work is not worth it. For whatever reasons they push on you, ignore them. *You are in the arena.*

That isn't to say you should avoid everyone.

There are people who will try to help you. In every crowd, there are true fans—people who want you to succeed. Those people are the ones you listen to. There will be people who have experienced what you're going through—the veterans and experienced mentors. These people will help you grow and direct you.

Not everyone is noise.

When my first medical practice was failing, I was fortunate to listen to an ex-clinic owner on what I was doing wrong. There was a sea of people telling me things that didn't help, but one person was trying to guide me. He was helping me succeed and to this day, I can't thank him enough. He showed me how to properly train staff, how to read contracts and encouraged me to take risks where possible.

Find out who is genuinely supporting you.

I have always wondered how amazing achievers deal with the noise. They are ridiculed by the media and shot down by haters. Some even get backstabbed by their best friends. Yet, they silence the haters and make the people who have ridiculed them for years shut up.

How?

By achieving their own goals. Once you achieve your goal, everything they have said about you—your poor form, your lack of effort—vanishes instantly.

How can people deny results? They can't. It's in their face.

So, what do you have to do?

Achieve it.

Build something first, and then talk about it. If you aren't comfortable having an audience, keep quiet and stay low.

Don't let anyone know, and work in silence. Many achievers have done so. I once loved telling people all my ideas, but throwing your ideas around blindly opens you up to criticism.

I told my friend about my idea to create a game company. He laughed it off, telling me it was stupid and a waste of time. Every day he told me that I should stop thinking about it and just concentrate on what I was good at. It definitely beat me down and I actually stopped pursuing it—till one day I said to myself, '*Fuck him. I'm going to do it anyway.*'

But this time, I chose to do it in silence.

I realized that nothing really changes if you tell people or you don't. *You pick the audience* that will support you. You curate the people that matter to you. The rest don't need to know anything.

You covertly work on your idea and, once it's finished, you release it. You show the world your results.

It can be tempting to show your progress, but the world doesn't care how far you have moved till you are near the end. People love chopping you down as you move along your journey, but once you're so close to the finish line, they can only support you. Otherwise, they look like the non-believer who got it wrong.

So, just achieve. The noise will fade with it.

31. YOU CHASE PASSION

"Follow your passion" sounds great.

Imagine finding something in your life that you love so much and get paid to do it. What a great dream. What a life that would be.

It sure sounds great, but how is that good advice? All of a sudden, the people who don't have a passion are left out? Who decided that passion should make you money?

The whole passion bullshit has got to stop. To achieve what you want, you *don't* follow your passion. You follow the path that helps you achieve what you want.

I have a friend who's an amazing engineer. He loves to modify old cars. He's passionate about it. It's pretty much the one thing he does in his free time. And if he could endlessly talk about one thing, it's cars.

But he gets paid a lot of money for his work. He's also really good at it. Like damn good at it. So why would he quit his work to follow his passion? His work gives him the money that allows him to work on cars.

Does he love his work? No.

Some days we can hate work. Some days we can enjoy it.

Like your passion, some days it can be the most stressful thing in your life; other days, it's what you want to do forever.

Don't get me wrong, some people have been fortunate to find their passion and get paid for it.

But what does my friend want to *achieve*? He wants to build a family. His passion won't do shit for that. His job will.

How many people do you know who have genuinely converted their passion to become their job? I can name only one personally. Does he love his work every day? No.

How many people can you name who work a job they are good at, while having a passion on the side? Plenty.

I know an accountant with a baking job on the weekends and a pharmacist with a wedding photography business. Are they happy? Yes. Are they making a lot of money from their passions? Not really.

I'm not saying you shouldn't *try* making your passion into your everyday job. I mean, why not? It would be ridiculous for me to tell you not to, but don't go quitting your day job for it.

Will you still enjoy your passion? Not sure. We all crave to be "that story": the person who quits their high paying job to follow their passion. Even I crave to be that story sometimes.

But is it realistic? No.

Even if it doesn't make you money, you can still love and enjoy your passion without the stress of it needing to be a money machine as well.

I met a popular YouTuber in Australia. I loved his videos; they were funny, and I always looked forward to next one. Making videos was his passion— and he wasn't making a bit of money from them. He just loved making people laugh and he released the videos whenever he felt like it.

As he got more popular, he realized he could make money from his passion. But this meant he needed to produce a certain amount of content to make enough money to survive. He would also need to create a schedule so he was consistently uploading videos. Plus, he had to contact sponsors to get more sources of income.

His passion was now turning into his job.

And that's when he started to hate making videos.

He ended up quitting YouTube at half a million subscribers (no small feat today!)

He went back to his normal job and now uploads videos only on the odd occasion. His account doesn't grow as much anymore but he's loving it. He only makes a small amount of money now and he doesn't have any sponsors. He's just enjoying his passion.

I'm not trying to scare you—honest. You might end up becoming one of those rare people whose passion makes them money and they love it! But consider this story as an emphasis on the fact that *there is absolutely nothing wrong with keeping a job you are good at and working on your passion on the side.*

So, you might ask, what about people who don't have a passion?

If you don't have one but feel *compelled* to have one, go do something random, look for something new to do. If you aren't trying something outside of your routine, you aren't looking hard enough. That, or it's right in front of your face.

I remember a friend who would go rock climbing after work. He told me he didn't have a passion. Every weekend he went climbing in the countryside. He told me that his life sucked because he didn't know what to do, didn't have a passion.

It was right in front of his face.

But one day, he broke his arm. He didn't go to work. And what was most upsetting to him? He couldn't climb. So, he went to the gym to work on his grip strength until he recovered.

Just remember: it's okay to not have a passion. You don't *need* one to achieve. If one comes, it comes. If it doesn't, so what?

Who gives a fuck if you don't have a passion? You don't!

Don't chase having a passion because you *feel* like you need one.

Don't believe your passion *has* to make you money.

PART IV

PUTTING IT ALL INTO PLACE

32. LET'S TIE IT ALL UP

It's all about *you*.

You are the most important person in your life. You are responsible for everything that happens to you. You are the person who controls what happens and what will happen. It's you, you, and you!

I have created a list of questions that I go through with frustrated achievers to help target the areas that you need to concentrate on. So, let's check them out:

1. Are you willing to take the shot?

Are you willing to do whatever it takes to achieve your goal?

You must measure the risks required and be willing to play the game—all the while knowing that you might lose. What risk tolerance do you have? Take fewer shots or no shots if you're comfortable with where you are. Take more shots if you can afford to do so. The bigger the goal, the more resources you must commit to making your shot count.

2. What are you complaining about?

What is it that is gnawing away at you every day? What are you complaining about the most? Target that first and address the problem. Not earning enough? Find ways to earn more. Maybe you want to become an influencer? Find ways to build your social media account.

Whatever your goal, answer and solve your complaints first.

3. Why are you procrastinating?

Remind yourself that life isn't certain. It's not about wasting all your money or shitting yourself that you may die tomorrow. Life is unpredictable and you never know when something (negative or positive) will happen in your life, so start your goals now.

You are betting against time, and time is a finite resource. Stop wasting it and start now.

4. What happened to your ambition?

You have *always* had aspirations. If you dream of something, that's ambition. Discard the things people have said that shot you down and the people who said you aren't capable. Remind yourself that you have a vision on where you want to be. Face that direction and go.

You are capable of acting on your ambition.

5. Are you scared to fail?

Failure is *part* of the process of succeeding. Accept that in order to achieve what you want you *must* fail. It's inevitable. But the most important part is taking the lessons you learn from your failures.

Each failure is a lesson, a lesson to help get you *closer* to your goal. Who wouldn't want to be closer to achieving their dreams?

6. What work-life balance do you need to achieve your goal?

Are you willing to put in the hours required to achieve what you want? If you don't have the time, where can you find more?

You may have to cut away some of your luxuries. You may have to reduce the time you get to enjoy life. Depending on what you want to achieve, your balance will vary. But be real with what you need and tweak your life in that direction.

7. Are you disciplined?

Remember: discipline is a muscle. It works in *all* facets in your life. You must work on it every day and it is a never-ending battle.

In order to achieve your goals, you need to remember that discipline keeps you on track. Whether it's the food you eat, the everyday chores you do, or the time you dedicate to your goals, discipline is the key component.

8. Do you have flashes of inspiration?

When you get a flash of inspiration, what do you do? You must act immediately on the extra energy inspiration gives you. Use that energy to help you get over obstacles preventing you from achieving your goals. You can write down your ideas in a book. You can call a friend and arrange a meeting. No matter what you do, don't waste your flashes of inspiration. They are rare moments that help you move closer to achieving your goals.

9. Are you already motivated?

You don't need much motivation to get started, but are you jumping from one motivational thing to another? Make sure you have a clear direction on where you are headed before you start filling your motivational tank.

Don't be addicted to motivation.

10. You say you don't have enough time

You do have time. You just don't have the right priorities. Do the 168-hour test to estimate how much time you have in your week. Then, start actively searching for ways you can find time. If wasted time doesn't show up in your estimate, trim time from other activities in your life. Otherwise, you won't achieve your goal.

11. Are you in a downswing?

Life is full of ups and downs. It is perfectly fine to be upset or angry. But to achieve your goals you must *minimize* the time you're in those downswings. You will end up wasting time—time better spent moving on to your next project, your next relationship or your next investment.

12. What is actually in your control?

When you're upset and wondering whether you can change something, ask yourself what, if any, parts are actually under your control. Any part that isn't under your control must be let go. If it's not in your control, you can't do anything about it, so why waste your time thinking about it?

Work only on what you can control.

13. Do you believe?

Do you believe you will achieve your goal? Do you see yourself getting what you desire? If you don't believe in yourself, you can't achieve anything. Without belief, you won't be able to get through the tough times. With belief, you can power through when shit hits the fan. Sometimes belief is the only thing you have.

14. Are you real with your goals?

What is the reason for your goal? Is it for the money? Personal achievement? Fame? Whatever the reason, be honest with yourself. The reason is yours and yours alone. It will make you tick and keep you moving. Be real and honest. There is no point lying to yourself.

15. Do you make your goals non-negotiable?

Your goals *are* non-negotiable. If you're serious on achieving what you want, you can't negotiate with the time you allocate to your goals. Friend calls you? Sorry, you're busy. Massive party coming? Too bad, you can't go. Allocate time and stick to it; otherwise, why did you make a plan to achieve?

16. Do you have a real deadline?

A goal is not complete unless you have a deadline. But a deadline also needs a consequence. Without that, you won't get it done. Be creative, ask a friend to make you responsible, make a bet on yourself. Or give up something if you don't achieve your goal by a certain date.

Set a deadline and a consequence.

17. Are you getting distracted?

Every distraction is your responsibility. If your phone is bothering you, it's your fault it's there. If the Internet browser is open, you opened it—which means you're responsible for closing it.

Whatever the distraction is, it is in your control to remove. So get rid of it.

18. Is your goal actually challenging you?

If something is easy, why bother doing it? Make your goal challenging, but within the realm of possibility. It's the goals that are challenging and exciting that will push you to your limits.

19. Can you tell me how far along you are and what's left?

You must break down your goal to quantifiable metrics as much as possible. The more you can measure, the better. If you want to increase your muscle mass, measure the actual size. If you want to improve your speed, why not time yourself?

Track your progress every time you work on your goals.

Stay motivated by looking at how far you have travelled and you how much further you have left to go. Measure everything you can.

20. Is it getting boring?

Well, tough luck. You have to deal with boring shit all the time. That's part of success. You can't ignore the boring stuff. Either do it or give up.

21. Are you firing on all cylinders?

Have you made the shot? Or are you simply stalling, hoping for the perfect plan?

You need to make the shot and adjust afterward.

Don't wait till you are perfect because it might be too late.

22. What have you actually finished?

You need to finish your goals. How many goals on your list have you done? Stay committed to the plan you made. Remind yourself that you didn't make a plan just to not complete it.

Finish what you start or don't even start at all.

23. Have you stopped caring about the small stuff?

Do you think the small things are too insignificant and not worth doing? Incremental steps, no matter how small, will help you achieve your goal. Everything starts with one. Learn one new word. Take one extra step. No matter what it may be, everything counts.

24. Are you craving for a magic bullet?

Shortcuts don't work. If they did, we would all be achievers. The larger the goal is, the longer it will take. Don't waste your time trying to find a shortcut.

We want to save as much time as possible to get what we want, but if we just look for a "quick" way around, we are simply wasting more time instead of just doing the damn hard work.

25. Can you stick to one goal?

Are you switching between goals? Are you jumping from one thing to another? Remind yourself you have only one goal at the top of your list. Priorities matter. One goal and one goal only.

26. Who are you comparing to?

Are you wasting time making comparisons? No comparison is fair. You have no idea about other people's pasts. You don't know what hard work they have been through.

The only person you should compare yourself to is yesterday's version of yourself.

27. Are you being selfish enough?

To achieve what you want, you must run on *your* clock, not someone else's. You have to be selfish with your time if you want to succeed with your goals. Your time is limited. Think carefully when using it for others. If you are unsure, use that time for you.

28. What or who is the toxic in your life?

You don't have the time for toxic people (or situations) in your life. Toxicity will prevent you from achieving your goals. Instead of burning the bridge, no longer maintain the relationship and see what unfolds. Toxicity will consume your mental space, your time, and your energy. If you have something toxic in your life, it must go. If you don't drop this toxic element, you will never obtain what you want.

29. Are you seeking revenge?

Success is the best revenge. Ignore and forget those who hurt or mistreated you. They are not worth your time. Learn from your mistakes and move on. Any time spent chasing revenge is not worthwhile. Use that energy to fuel your next positive move, whether it's your next idea or business plan.

30. Are the people around you helping you?

Do you have a mentor or someone to guide you to achieve your goal? Is there noise that is trying to pull you down? Think carefully of those who are around you and who have been supportive. No journey has to be alone. Find the people who are supporting you and build a relationship. Ask them for guidance.

The criticizers? Silence them with your achievement.

31. Are you chasing passion?

You don't need to chase your passion. Chase what you are good at to fuel your passion on the side. Don't ever think you are failing because you don't have a passion. There's nothing wrong with not having one.

Don't chase passion.

So, what areas resonated with you?

To achieve your goals, concentrate on what you can achieve. Remember, this book revolves around *you*, your goals, your surroundings—everything that is within your control.

Now, with that said....

33. GO ACHIEVE YOUR GOAL ALREADY

So, what happened to Terry? Remember him from the "Frustrated Achievers" prologue? He quit his job. He always wanted to run his own investment firm. Instead of partying and playing computer games, he actually spent time working on his business idea. He stopped caring about the toxic people in his life.

His boss still treated him like crap. His friends still asked him to go out.

He noticed that even when he stopped caring about the relationships that were cruel to him, nothing really changed.

He stayed in these relationships because he always felt he never belonged and wanted people to like him. He started to care for himself and work on what he wanted. No longer was he wasting time with shit that didn't matter. It was all on him now.

For Terry, the most fundamental change was his internal belief that he couldn't do it. He knew exactly what needed to be done but just couldn't commit himself.

When he would tell people his ideas, they would shoot them down. Over time, he no longer believed in himself. He let the world crush his dreams and goals. He settled with what he had and instead would complain to people who would listen to him (myself included!). He whined—and then went back to work. Rinse and repeat. It finally clicked that his friends were toxic. He realized that he could do what he wanted if he tried. *Truth is: He could always do it.*

Before I finished this book, I met with Terry one more time. He came with his wife and he was damn happy. It had been four years since that first talk. He owns a small boutique investment firm and has a child.

"You know, man, we had a holiday in Maldives." was his opening line—miles away from a paraphrased version of "I hate my work."

We ended up talking about general life stuff. I have no doubt he went through a whole lot of shit to get to where he is today including the fact that his old company tried to sue him or even the temptations to go back to a routine life.

But he made it. *He freaking made it!*

He achieved what he wanted.

I knew he could, but I am in no position to tell him that. Everyone has to figure it out for themselves.

What I hope you get from this book is that you were always capable of achieving what you want. The shit that stops us is in our control. Don't ever forget that. So, what are you waiting for? The path to achieving what you want will take a long damn time—or, if you are lucky—less than a long damn time.

You need to go now. Fuck the motivating words.

You know you can do it.

Go.

Just fucking achieve.

ACKNOWLEDGMENTS

I dedicate this book to all those frustrated achievers out there.

To the ones I met, thank you for your stories and your time. I hope you achieve the shit you are capable of, because for fuck's sake, you *are*. *You deserve to have what you want.*

Thank you to Maria, for your ongoing support and guidance through the world of publishing. Thank you to Nina for helping me improve this book and making it the best version it can be.

And thank *you*.

You made this book possible.

You have always been at the core of this book.

You, the person who should be achieving far more than they have so far.

You, the person who now will be on the path to your dreams.

www.ingramcontent.com/pod-product-compliance
Lightning Source LLC
Chambersburg PA
CBHW032146020426

42334CB00016B/1245

* 9 7 8 0 6 4 8 9 1 3 5 2 8 *